Essentials of Hospital Finance

William O. Cleverley, Ph.D.

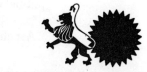

AN ASPEN PUBLICATION®
Aspen Systems Corporation
Rockville, Maryland
Royal Tunbridge Wells
1978

Library of Congress Cataloging in Publication Data

Cleverley, William O.

Essentials of hospital finance.

Includes index.
1. Hospitals—Finance. 2. Hospitals—Accounting.
I. Title. [DNLM: 1. Financial management.
2. Economics, Hospital. WX157.3 C635e]

RA971.3.C53   658.1'5932   78-7447
ISBN 0-89443-035-1

Library of Congress Catalog Card Number: 78-7447
ISBN: 0-89443-035-1

Printed in the United States of America

7   8   9   10

To My Students

Table of Contents

Foreword

Dr. Cleverley has presented a well-written, informative and particularly needed "how-to" book. A quick review of the Table of Contents and you will recognize it is designed for almost anyone who needs to better understand hospital finance. This includes hospital departmental managers, administrators and governing boards with internal operating or policy responsibilities. It certainly can be helpful to health planning agency personnel, Blue Cross and commercial insurance or other third-party payer personnel, bankers, and auditors or accountants who have not had previous hospital experience.

One of the most difficult areas for a young health administrator to master and in which to obtain satisfactory experience is finance. I suspect it is because financial management is an extremely critical aspect of the total overall hospital operation, and often retained by the senior operations officer. As a result, many otherwise extremely competent young managers become Chief Executive Officers responsible for a rather sizable operation and may not feel comfortable in the area of finance. For them, this book can be most helpful.

The definitions of financial terms and the explanation of the purposes of the four basic financial statements are included, along with financial ratios. Continuous review of the ratios and ratio trends are a vitally important part of prudent financial planning. Although scarcely discussed a few years ago, today they are the "report cards" by which bankers or other lending agencies (and often one's own governing board) will evaluate the strength and financial potential of an institution.

Effective resource utilization is a basic element of good management. It requires the hospital finance officer to have the tools available for adequate counseling to management in both the planning process and in the deadly serious game of "what-if?" This book provides the formulas for many of these important calculations. In summary, Dr. Cleverley has added an important book to my armamentarium as a health care manager.

Wade Mountz
May 1978

Preface

The idea for this book originated from a series of adult education programs conducted for health care managers, health care financing specialists, health systems agency staff and hospital boards of trustees. In almost every situation these individuals evidenced a critical need to understand the meaning and relevance of financial information and financial management in the health care industry to adequately perform their assigned responsibilities. However, few had prior knowledge of accounting or financial management as it is practiced in the health care industry. Because of their existing commitments, they neither had the time nor the interest to correct this situation.

This book is an attempt to provide a remedy for this situation. It provides for a discussion of the principles of health care accounting and financial management. Unlike many textbooks in accounting or finance, there is no presumption of any prerequisite knowledge in accounting, finance or economics. In addition, a glossary of terms has been included to explain much of the jargon used in the health care industry.

The ultimate objective of this book is to improve the understanding and use of financial information by decision makers in the health care industry. Informed and intelligent use of financial information in the health care industry is no longer a luxury but a necessity of the most basic sort.

Many individuals were instrumental in the development and completion of this book. First, I credit the many adult education students who not only impressed upon me the need to write this book, but also served as a critical review group for much of the material contained herein. Secondly, Dr. Robert Caswell of The Ohio State University provided key editorial comments that unquestionably enhanced the readability of this book. Third, Ms. Joan Wilson in her consistent efficient manner typed, retyped and reviewed the entire contents of this manuscript. Finally, I wish to acknowledge the patience and understanding of my wife, Linda, and our three children, Michelle, Meredith and Jamie.

Chapter 1

Financial Information and the Decision-Making Process

This book is intended to improve decision makers' understanding and use of financial information in the health care industry. It is not an advanced treatise in accounting or finance but an elementary discussion of how financial information in general, and health care industry financial information in particular, are interpreted and used. It is written for individuals who are not experienced health care financial executives—to make the language of health care finance readable and relevant for general decision makers in the health care industry.

Three interdependent factors have created the need for this book:

1. rapid expansion of the health care industry;
2. health care decision maker's general lack of business and financial background;
3. financial and cost criteria's increasing importance in health care decisions.

The health care industry's rapid expansion is a trend visible even to individuals outside the health care system: the hospital industry, the major component of the health care industry, is consuming an increasing portion of the Gross National Product; other types of health care systems, though smaller than the hospital industry, are expanding at even faster rates. Exhibit 1-1 lists the types of major health care institutions and indexes their relative size.

The rapid growth of health care facilities providing direct medical services has substantially increased the number of decision makers who need to be familiar with financial information; even greater expansion in the number of decision makers indirectly involved in health care has compounded the need. Most of these decision makers work with health care regulations. Effective decision making in their jobs

1

depends on an accurate interpretation of financial information. Many health care decision makers involved directly in health care delivery—doctors, nurses, dieticians, pharmacists, radiation technologists, physical therapists, inhalation therapists—are medically or scientifically trained but lack education and experience in business and finance. Their specialized education, in most cases, did not include such courses as accounting. However, advancement and promotion within health care organizations increasingly entails assumption of administrative duties, requiring almost instant knowledgeable reading of financial information. Communication with the organization's financial executives is not always helpful. As a result, nonfinancial executives often end up ignoring financial information.

Governing boards, significant users of financial information, are expanding in size in many health care facilities, in some cases to accommodate demands for more consumer representation. This trend can be healthy for both the community and the facilities. However, many board members, even those with backgrounds in business, are being overwhelmed by financial reports and statements. There are important distinctions between the financial statements of business organizations (with which some board members are familiar) and those of health care facilities which governing board members must recognize to carry out their governing mission satisfactorily.

Decision makers involved in regulation have also multiplied. These decision makers work primarily with quantitative information provided by the facilities they regulate; most of this information is financial, especially in planning agencies (health systems agencies) and rate regulatory commissions. Many of these very important and influential decision makers have some background in accounting and finance, but it may not be sufficient for their assigned tasks. In most situations the agency staff only serve as a source of input for decisions that are made by a governing board. These boards usually represent a public constituency and may have little or no understanding and experience with financial data. It is highly important for these individuals to have some minimum level of financial awareness if effective regulatory decisions are to be made.

The increasing importance of financial and cost criteria in health care decision making is the third factor which creates a need for more knowledge of financial information. For many years, accountants and financial people have been caricatured as individuals with narrow vision, incapable of seeing the forest for the trees. In many respects, this may have been an accurate portrayal. However, few individuals in the health care industry today would deny the importance of financial concerns, especially cost. Careful attention to these concerns requires *knowledgeable* consumption of financial information by a variety of decision makers. It is not an overstatement to say that inattention to financial criteria can lead to excessive costs and eventually to insolvency.

INFORMATION AND DECISION MAKING

The major function of information in general, and financial information in particular, is to oil the decision-making process. Decision making is basically the selection of a course of action from a defined list of possible or feasible actions. In many cases, the actual course of action followed may be essentially no action—decision makers may decide to make no change from their present policies. It should be recognized that action or no action represents a policy decision.

Exhibit 1-2 illustrates how information is related to the decision-making process and gives an example to illustrate the sequence. Generating information is the key to decision-making. The quality and effectiveness of decision making depends on accurate, timely, relevant information. It is important to note that the difference between data and information is more than semantic: data becomes information *only* when it is useful and appropriate to the decision. Much financial data never becomes information because it is not viewed as relevant or is unavailable in an intelligent form.

For the illustrative purposes of the burn care unit example in Exhibit 1-2, only two possible courses of action are assumed: to build or not build a burn care unit. In most situations there may be a continuum of alternative courses of action. For example, a burn care unit might be varied by bed size or facilities included in the unit. Prior decision making seems to have reduced the feasible set of alternatives to a more manageable and limited number for analysis.

Once a course of action has been selected in the decision-making phase, it must be accomplished. Implementing a decision may be extremely complex. In the burn care unit example, carrying out the decision to build the unit would require enormous management effort to insure that the projected results are actually obtained. Periodic measurement of results in a feedback loop (Exhibit 1-2) is a method commonly used to make sure that decisions are actually implemented according to pre-established plans.

As previously stated, results that are forecast are not always guaranteed. Controllable factors, such as failure to adhere to prescribed plans, and uncontrollable circumstances such as a change in reimbursement may obstruct planned results.

Decision making usually takes place in uncertainty. No anticipated result of a decision is guaranteed. Events may occur which have been analyzed but not anticipated. A results matrix concisely portrays the possible results of various courses of action, given the occurrence of possible events; Exhibit 1-3 provides a results matrix for the sample burn care unit; it shows that approximately 50% utilization will enable this unit to operate in the black and not drain resources from other areas. If forecasting shows that utilization below 50% is unlikely, decision makers may very well elect to build.

A good information system should enable decision makers to choose courses of action with the most highly expected results. Based on the results matrix of Exhibit 3 a good information system should specifically—

1. list possible courses of action;
2. list possible events which might occur, affecting the expected results;
3. indicate the probability of those events occurring;
4. accurately estimate the results given an action/event combination (e.g., profit in Exhibit 1-3).

One thing an information system does not do is evaluate the desirability of results. Decision makers must evaluate results in terms of their organizations' or their own preferences. For example, construction of a burn care unit may be expected to lose $200,000 a year, but it could save a significant number of lives. Weighing these results, or criteria, is purely a decision maker's responsibility—not an easy task, but one that can be improved with accurate and relevant information.

USES AND USERS OF FINANCIAL INFORMATION

As a subset of information in general, financial information is important in the decision-making process. In some areas of decision making financial information is especially relevant. For our purposes we will identify five uses of financial information that may be important in decision making:

1. evaluating the *financial condition* of an entity;
2. evaluating *stewardship* within an entity;
3. assessing the *efficiency* of operations;
4. assessing the *effectiveness* of operations;
5. determining the *compliance* of operations with directives.

Financial Condition

Of these five areas, evaluating an entity's financial condition is probably the most common use of financial information. Usually, an organization's financial condition is equated with its viability or capacity to continue pursuing its stated goals at a consistent level of activity. However, viability is a far less restrictive term than solvency. Some health care organizations may be solvent but not viable. For example, a hospital may have its level of funds restricted so that it must reduce its scope of activity but still remain solvent. A reduction in approved rates by a designated regulatory or rate selling agency may be the vehicle for this change in viability.

Assessing the financial condition of business enterprises is essential to our economy's smooth and efficient operation. Most business decisions in our economy are directly or indirectly based on perceptions of financial condition. This includes the largely nonprofit health care industry. Though attention is usually directed at organizations as whole units, assessing the financial condition of organizational divisions is equally important. In the burn unit example, the future financial condition of the unit is valuable. If continued losses from this operation are projected, impairment of the financial condition of other divisions in the organization could be in the offing.

Assessing financial condition also includes consideration of short-run versus long-run effects. The relevant time frame may change depending on the decision under consideration. For example, suppliers are typically interested only in an organization's short-run financial condition because that is the period in which they must expect payment. However, investment bankers, as long-term creditors, are interested in the organization's financial condition over a much longer time period.

Stewardship

Historically, evaluating stewardship was the most important use of accounting and financial information systems. These systems were originally designed to prevent the loss of assets or resources through employees' malfeasance. Their use is still very important. The relatively infrequent occurrence of employee fraud and embezzlement may be due in part to the deterrence of well designed accounting systems.

Efficiency

Efficiency in health care operations is becoming an increasingly important objective for many decision makers. Efficiency is simply the ratio of outputs to inputs, not the quality of outputs—good or not good—but the lowest possible cost of production. Adequate assessment of efficiency implies the availability of a standard against which actual costs may be compared. In many health care organizations, these standards may be formally introduced into the budgetary process. For example, a given nursing unit may have an efficiency standard of 4.3 nursing hours per patient day of care delivered. This standard may then be used as a benchmark to evaluate the relative efficiency within the unit. For example, actual employment of six nursing hours per patient day may cause management to assess staffing patterns.

Effectiveness

Assessment of the effectiveness of operations is concerned with the attainment of objectives through production of outputs, not the relationship of outputs to cost. Measuring effectiveness is much more difficult than measuring efficiency because most organizations' objectives or goals are typically not stated quantitatively. Because measurement is difficult, there is a tendency to place less emphasis on effectiveness and more on efficiency. This may result in the delivery of unneeded services at an efficient cost. For example, development of outpatient surgical centers may reduce costs per surgical procedure and thus create an efficient means of delivery. However, the necessity of those surgical procedures may still be questionable.

Compliance

Finally, financial information may be used to determine whether compliance with directives has taken place. The best example of an organization's internal directives is its budget, an agreement between two management levels regarding use of resources for a defined time period. External parties may also impose directives for the organization's adherence, many of them financial in nature. For example, rate setting or regulatory agencies may set limits on rates determined within an organization. Financial reporting by the organization is required to ensure compliance.

Exhibit 1-4 presents a matrix of users and uses of financial information in the health care industry. It exemplifies areas or uses that may interest particular decision-making groups. It does not consider relative importance.

Not every use of financial information is important in every decision. For example, in approving a health care organization's rates, a governing board may be interested in only two uses of financial information: assessment of financial condition and assessment of operational efficiency. Other uses may be irrelevant. The board wants to ensure that services are being provided efficiently and that sufficient rates are being established to guarantee a stable or improved financial condition. As Exhibit 1-4 illustrates, health care decision-making groups mostly use financial information to assess financial condition and efficiency. This book will discuss what specific types of financial information are used to make these assessments and how this information is interpreted.

Exhibit 1-1 Health Care Expenditures, 1974–1976 (In Millions)

	1974	1976	Percentage Change
Total Expenditures	$106,321	$139,312	34.8%
Hospital Care	41,020	55,400	35.1
Physicians' Services	19,742	26,350	33.5
Dentists' Services	6,870	8,600	25.2
Other Professional Services	1,929	2,400	24.4
Drugs & Drug Sundries	9,416	11,168	18.6
Eyeglasses & Appliances	1,674	1,980	18.3
Nursing Home Care	7,450	10,600	42.3
Other Health Services	3,214	3,933	22.4
Prepayment & Administration	5,483	7,336	33.8
Government Public Health Activities	2,531	3,255	28.6
Research and Construction	6,991	8,290	18.6

Exhibit 1-2 Information in the Decision-Making Process

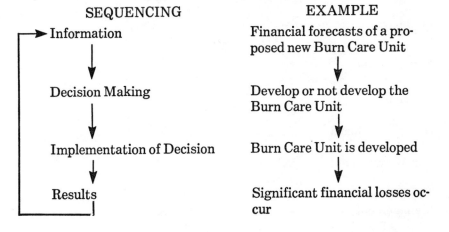

SEQUENCING	EXAMPLE
Information	Financial forecasts of a proposed new Burn Care Unit
Decision Making	Develop or not develop the Burn Care Unit
Implementation of Decision	Burn Care Unit is developed
Results	Significant financial losses occur

Exhibit 1-3 Results Matrix/Burn Care Example

Alternative Actions	EVENT		
	25% Utilization	50% Utilization	75% Utilization
Build Unit	$400,000 Loss	$10,000 Profit	$200,000 Profit
Do Not Build Unit	0	0	0

Exhibit 1-4 Users and Uses of Financial Information

Users	USES				
	Financial Condition	Steward-ship	Effi-ciency	Effective-ness	Com-pliance
External					
Health System Agencies	X		X	X	X
Unions	X		X		
Rate Setting Organizations	X		X	X	X
Creditors	X		X	X	
Third Party Payers			X		X
Suppliers	X				
Public	X		X	X	
Internal					
Governing Board	X	X	X	X	X
Top Management	X	X	X	X	X
Departmental Management			X		X

Chapter 2

General Principles of Accounting

Information does not happen by itself; it must be generated by an individual or a formally designed system. Financial information is no exception. The accounting system generates most financial information to provide quantitative data primarily financial in nature that is useful in making economic decisions about economic entities.

FINANCIAL VERSUS MANAGERIAL ACCOUNTING

Financial accounting is the branch of accounting which provides general purpose financial statements or reports to aid a large number of decision-making groups, internal and external to the organization, in a variety of decisions. The primary outputs of financial accounting are four financial statements that will be discussed in Chapter 3:

- Balance Sheet
- Statement of Revenues and Expenses
- Statement of Changes in Financial Position
- Statement of Changes in Fund Balance

Examples of these four financial statements are contained in Exhibits 3-1, 3-2, 3-3, 3-4 and 3-5.

The field of financial accounting is restricted in many ways regarding how certain events or business transactions may be accounted for. The term "generally accepted accounting principles" is often used to describe the body of rules and requirements that shape the preparation of the four primary financial statements. For example, an organization's financial statements that have been audited by an independent certified public accountant (CPA) bear the following language:

> In our opinion, the aforementioned financial statements present fairly the financial position of the XYZ Company at December 31, 1978 and the results of its operations and changes in its financial position for the year ended in conformity with generally accepted accounting principles applied on a basis consistent with that of the preceding year.

Financial accounting is not limited to preparation of the four statements. An increasing number of additional financial reports are being required, especially for external users in specific decision-making purposes. This is particularly important in the health care industry. For example, hospitals submit cost reports to a number of third party payers such as Blue Cross, Medicare, and Medicaid. They also submit financial reports to a large number of regulatory agencies, such as planning agencies, rate review agencies, service associations and many others. These statements, while not usually audited by independent CPAs are, for the most part, prepared in accordance with the same generally accepted accounting principles that govern the preparation of the four basic financial statements.

Managerial accounting is primarily concerned with the preparation of financial information for specific purposes, usually for internal users. Since this information is used within the organization, there is less need for a body of principles restricting its preparation. Presumably, the user and the preparer can meet to discuss questions of interpretation. Uniformity and comparability of information, which are desired goals for financial accountants, are clearly less important to management accountants.

PRINCIPLES OF ACCOUNTING

This book focuses on both sets of accounting information, financial and managerial. While managerial accounting has no formally adopted set of principles, it relies strongly on financial accounting principles. Understanding the principles and basics of financial accounting is therefore critical to understanding both financial and managerial accounting information.

The case example for our discussion of the principles of financial accounting will be a newly formed, nonprofit community hospital which shall be referred to as "Alpha Hospital."

Accounting Entity

It is not too obvious to mention that in any accounting there must be an entity for which financial statements are being prepared.

Specifying the entity upon which the accounting will focus defines what information is pertinent. Drawing these boundaries is the underlying concept behind the accounting entity principle.

Alpha Hospital will be the entity for which we will account and prepare financial statements. We are not interested in the individuals who may have incorporated Alpha or other hospitals in the community, but solely in Alpha Hospital's financial transactions.

Defining the entity is not as clear-cut as one might expect. Significant problems arise, especially when the legal entity is different from the accounting entity. For example, if one doctor owns a clinic through a sole proprietorship arrangement, the accounting entity may be the clinic operation while the legal entity includes the doctor and the doctor's personal resources as well. Or for example, a hospital may be part of a university or government agency, or it might be owned by a large corporation organized on a profit or nonprofit basis. Careful attention must be paid to the definition of the accounting entity in these situations. If the entity is not properly defined, evaluation of its financial information may be useless at best, and misleading at worst.

The common practice of municipalities directly paying the fringe benefits of municipal employees employed in the hospital illustrates this situation. Such expenses may never show up in the hospital's accounts, resulting in an understatement of the expenses associated with running the hospital, and in many cases, a reduction in the absolute level of reimbursement to which the organization is entitled.

Money Measurement

Accounting in general, but financial accounting in particular, is concerned with measuring economic resources and obligations and their changing levels for the accounting entity under consideration. The accountant's yardstick for measuring is not metered to size, color, weight or other attributes but is limited exclusively to money. There are significant problems in money measurement which will be discussed shortly.

Economic resources are defined as scarce means, limited in supply but essential to economic activity. They include supplies, buildings, equipment, money, claims to receive money and ownership interests in other enterprises. The terms *economic resources* and *assets* may be interchanged for most practical purposes. Economic obligations are responsibilities to transfer economic resources or provide services to other entities in the future, usually in return for economic resources received from other entities in the past through the purchase of assets, the receipt of services or the acceptance of loans. For most practical purposes, the terms economic obligations and liabilities may be used interchangeably.

In most normal situations, assets exceed liabilities in money measured value. Liabilities represent the claim of one entity on another's assets; any excess, or remaining residual interest, may be claimed by the owner. In fact, for entities with ownership interest, this residual interest is called "owner's equity."

In most nonprofit entities, including health care organizations, there is no residual ownership claim. Any assets remaining in a liquidated not-for-profit entity, after all liabilities have been dissolved, legally become the property of the state. Residual interest is referred to as "fund balance" for most health care organizations.

For the Alpha Hospital example, assume that the community donated $1 million in cash to the hospital at its formation, hypothetically assumed to be December 31, 1977. At that time, a listing of its assets, liabilities and fund balance would be prepared in a balance sheet and read as below:

ALPHA HOSPITAL
BALANCE SHEET
December 31, 1977

Assets	Liabilities and Fund Balance
Cash $1,000,000	Fund Balance $1,000,000

Duality

One of the fundamental premises of accounting is a very simple arithmetic requirement: the value of assets must always equal the combined value of liabilities and residual interest, which we have called fund balance. This basic accounting equation, the *duality principle,* may be stated as follows:

$$\text{Assets} = \text{Liabilities} + \text{Fund Balance}$$

This requirement means that a balance sheet will always balance— the value of the assets will always equal the value of claims whether liabilities or fund balance, on those assets.

Changes are always occurring in organizations which affect the value of assets, liabilities and fund balance. These changes are called transactions and represent the items which interest accountants. Examples of transactions include borrowing money, purchasing supplies and constructing buildings. The important thing to remember is that each transaction must be carefully analyzed under the duality principle to keep the basic accounting equation in balance.

To better understand how important this principle is, let us analyze several transactions for the Alpha Hospital example.

Transaction No. 1
On January 2, 1978, Alpha Hospital buys a piece of equipment for $100,000. The purchase is financed with a $100,000 note from the bank.

Transaction No. 2
On January 3, 1978, Alpha Hospital buys a building for $2,000,000 using $500,000 cash and issuing $1,500,000 worth of 20-year bonds.

Transaction No. 3
On January 4, 1978, Alpha Hospital purchases $200,000 of supplies from a supply firm on a credit basis.

If balance sheets were prepared after each of the three transactions they would appear as follows:

ALPHA HOSPITAL
BALANCE SHEET
January 2, 1978

Assets		Liabilities and Fund Balance	
Cash	$1,000,000	Notes Payable	$100,000
Equipment	100,000	Fund Balance	1,000,000
TOTAL	$1,100,000	TOTAL	$1,100,000

Assets: Increase $100,000 (Equipment increases by $100,000)
Liabilities: Increase $100,000 (Notes payable increase by $100,000)

ALPHA HOSPITAL
BALANCE SHEET
January 3, 1978

Assets		Liabilities and Fund Balance	
Cash	$ 500,000	Notes Payable	$ 100,000
Equipment	100,000	Bonds Payable	1,500,000
Building	2,000,000	Fund Balance	1,000,000
TOTAL	$2,600,000	TOTAL	$2,600,000

Assets: Increase $1,500,000 (Cash decreases by $500,000 and building increases by $2,000,000)
Liabilities: Increase $1,500,000 (Bonds payable increase by $1,500,000)

ALPHA HOSPITAL
BALANCE SHEET
January 4, 1978

Assets		Liabilities and Fund Balance	
Cash	$ 500,000	Accounts Payable	$ 200,000
Supplies	200,000	Notes Payable	• 100,000
Equipment	100,000	Bonds Payable	1,500,000
Building	2,000,000	Fund Balance	1,000,000
TOTAL	$2,800,000	TOTAL	$2,800,000

Assets: Increase $200,000 (Supplies increase by $200,000)
Liabilities: Increase $200,000 (Accounts payable increase by $200,000)

In each transaction, the change in asset value is matched by an identical change in liability value. Thus, the basic accounting equation remains in balance.

It should be noted that as the number of transactions increases, the number of individual asset and liability items also increase. In most organizations there is a very large number of these individual items which are referred to as accounts. The listing of these accounts is often called a chart of accounts; it is a useful device for categorizing transactions related to a given health care organization. There is already significant uniformity among hospitals and other health care facilities in the chart of accounts used, however, there is pressure, especially from external users of financial information, to move towards even more uniformity.

Cost Valuation

Many readers of financial statements make the mistake of assuming that reported balance sheet values represent the real worth of individual assets or liabilities. Asset and liability values reported in a balance sheet are based on their historical or acquisition cost. In most situations asset values do not equal the amount of money that could be realized if the assets were sold. However, in many cases the reported value of a liability in a balance sheet is a good approximation of the amount of money that would be required to extinguish the indebtedness.

Examining the alternatives to historical cost valuation helps clarify why the cost basis of valuation is used. The two primary alternatives to historical cost valuation of assets and liabilities are Market Value and Replacement Cost valuation.

Valuation of individual assets at their market value sounds simple enough and appeals to many users of financial statements. Creditors are often especially interested in what values assets would bring if liquidated. Current market values give decision makers an approximation of liquidation values.

The market value method's lack of objectivity is a serious problem. In most normal situations, established markets dealing in second hand merchandise do not exist. Decision makers must rely on individual appraisals. Given the current state of the art of appraisal, two appraisers are likely to produce different estimates of market value for an identical asset. Accountants' insistence on objectivity in measurement thus eliminates market valuation of assets as a viable alternative.

Replacement cost valuation of assets measures assets by the money value required to replace them. This concept of valuation is extremely useful for many decision making purposes. For example, management decisions to continue delivery of certain services should be affected by the replacement cost of resources, not their historical or acquisition cost—which is considered to be a sunk cost, irrelevant to future decisions. Planning agencies or other regulatory agencies should also consider incorporating estimates of replacement cost into their decisions to avoid bias. Considering only historical cost may improperly make old facilities appear more efficient than new or proposed facilities and projects.

While replacement cost may be a useful concept of valuation, it too suffers from lack of objectivity in measurement. Replacement cost valuation depends upon *how* an item is replaced. For example, given the rate of technological change in the general economy, especially in the health care industry, few assets of today would be replaced with like assets. Instead, more refined or capable assets would probably be substituted. What is the replacement cost in this situation? Is it the cost of the new, improved asset or the present cost of an identical asset that would most likely *not* be purchased? Compound this question by the large number of manufacturers selling roughly equivalent items and you have some idea of the inherent difficulty and subjectivity in replacement cost valuation.

Historical cost valuation, with all its faults, is the basis that the accounting profession has chosen to value assets and liabilities in most usual circumstances. Accountants use it in place of replacement cost largely because it is more objective. There is currently some fairly strong pressure from inside and outside the accounting profession to switch to replacement cost valuation, but it is still uncertain whether this movement will succeed.

One final, important point should be noted. At the time of initial asset valuation, the values assigned by historical cost valuation and replacement cost valuation are identical. The historical cost value is most often criticized for assets that have long useful lives, such as building and equipment. Over a period of many years, the historical cost and replacement cost values tend to diverge dramatically, partly because general inflation in our economy erodes the dollar's purchasing power. A dollar of today is simply not as valuable as a dollar of ten years ago. This problem could be remedied without sacrificing the objectivity of historical cost measurement by selecting a unit of purchasing power as the unit of measure: Transactions would not be accounted in dollars but in dollars of purchasing power at a given point in time, usually the year for which the financial statements are being prepared. We will discuss this issue later when we talk about the stable monetary unit principle.

Accrual Accounting

Accrual accounting is a fundamental premise of accounting which means that transactions of a business enterprise are recognized in the time period to which they relate and not necessarily in the time periods in which cash is received or paid.

It is quite common to hear people talk about an accrual versus a cash basis of accounting. Most of us think in cash basis terms. We measure our personal, financial success during the year by how much cash we took in. Very seldom do we consider such things as wear and tear on our cars and other personal items, or differences between earned and uncollected income. Perhaps if we accrued expenses for items like depreciation on heating systems, air conditioning systems, automobiles, and furniture, we might see a different picture of our financial well-being.

The accrual basis of accounting significantly affects the preparation of financial statements in general, however, its major impact is on the preparation of the Statement of Revenues and Expenses. The following additional transactions for Alpha Hospital illustrate the importance of the accrual principle.

Transaction No. 4
Alpha Hospital bills patients $100,000 on January 16, 1978, for services provided to them.

Transaction No. 5
Alpha Hospital pays employees $60,000 for their wages and salaries on January 18, 1978.

Transaction No. 6
Alpha Hospital receives $80,000 in cash from patients who were billed earlier in Transaction No. 4 on January 23, 1978.

Transaction No. 7
Alpha Hospital pays the $200,000 of Accounts Payable on January 27, 1978, for the purchase of supplies that took place on January 4, 1978.

Balance sheets prepared after each of the preceeding transactions would appear as follows:

ALPHA HOSPITAL
BALANCE SHEET
January 16, 1978

Assets		Liabilities and Fund Balance	
Cash	$500,000	Accounts Payable	$200,000
Accounts Receivable	100,000	Notes Payable	100,000
Supplies	200,000	Bonds Payable	1,500,000
Equipment	100,000	Fund Balance	1,100,000
Building	2,000,000		
TOTAL	$2,900,000	TOTAL	$2,900,000

Assets: Increase $100,000 (Accounts receivable increase by $100,000)
Fund Balance: Increases $100,000

ALPHA HOSPITAL
BALANCE SHEET
January 18, 1978

Assets		Liabilities and Fund Balance	
Cash	$440,000	Accounts Payable	$200,000
Accounts Receivable	100,000	Notes Payable	100,000
Supplies	200,000	Bonds Payable	1,500,000
Equipment	100,000	Fund Balance	1,040,000
Building	2,000,000		
TOTAL	$2,840,000	TOTAL	$2,840,000

Assets: Decrease by $60,000 (Cash decreases by $60,000)
Fund Balance: Decreases by $60,000

ALPHA HOSPITAL
BALANCE SHEET
January 23, 1978

Assets		Liabilities and Fund Balance	
Cash	$520,000	Accounts Payable	$200,000
Accounts Receivable	20,000	Notes Payable	100,000
Supplies	200,000	Bonds Payable	1,500,000
Equipment	100,000	Fund Balance	1,040,000
Building	2,000,000		
TOTAL	$2,840,000	TOTAL	$2,840,000

Assets: No Change (Cash increases by $80,000; accounts receivable
        decrease by $80,000)

ALPHA HOSPITAL
BALANCE SHEET
January 27, 1978

Assets		Liabilities and Fund Balance	
Cash	$320,000	Accounts Payable $	0
Accounts Receivable	20,000	Notes Payable	100,000
Supplies	200,000	Bonds Payable	1,500,000
Equipment	100,000	Fund Balance	1,040,000
Building	2,000,000		
TOTAL	$2,640,000	TOTAL	$2,640,000

Assets: Decrease by $200,000 (Cash decreases by $200,000)
Liabilities: Decrease by $200,000 (Accounts payable decrease by $200,000)

In the first two transactions, there is an effect upon Alpha Hospital's residual interest or its fund balance. In the first case, an increase in fund balance occurred due to the billing of patients for services previously rendered. Increases in fund balance or owner's equity resulting from the sale of goods or delivery of services are called revenues. It should be noted that this increase occurred even though no cash was actually collected until January 23, 1978, illustrating the accrual principle of accounting. Recognition of revenue occurs when the revenue is earned, not necessarily when it is collected.

In Transaction No. 5, a reduction in fund balance occurs. Costs incurred by a business enterprise to provide goods or services that reduce fund balance or owner's equity, are called expenses. Under the accrual principle, expenses are recognized when assets are used up or liabilities incurred in the production and delivery of goods or services, not necessarily when cash is paid.

The difference between revenue and expense is often referred to as net income. In the hospital and health care industry, this term may be used interchangeably with the term "excess of revenues over expenses."

The Income Statement or Statement of Revenues and Expenses summarizes the revenues and expenses of a business enterprise over a defined period of time. If an income statement is prepared for the total life of an entity, i.e. from inception to dissolution, it happens that the value for net income would be the same under both an accrual and a cash basis of accounting.

In most situations, frequent measurements of revenue and expense are demanded, creating some important measurement problems. Ideally, under the accrual accounting principle, expenses should be matched to the revenue which they helped create. For example, wage, salary and supply costs can usually be easily associated with revenues of a given period. However, in certain circumstances the association between revenue and expense is impossible to discover, necessitating the accountant's use of a systematic, rational method of allocating costs to a benefitting time period. In the best example of this procedure, costs such as those associated with building and equipment are spread over the estimated useful life of the assets through the recording of depreciation (see Glossary). George O. May, an accounting theorist, best summarizes this dilemma when he states, "The measurement of periodic net income would be indefensible if it were not indispensable."

To complete the Alpha Hospital example, we will assume that the financial statements must be prepared at the end of January. Before they may be prepared, certain adjustments must be made to the accounts to adhere fully to the accrual principle of accounting. The following adjustments might be recorded:

- *Adjustment No. 1*
  There are currently $100,000 of patient charges that have been incurred but not yet billed.
- *Adjustment No. 2*
  There is currently $50,000 worth of unpaid wages and salaries for which employees have performed services.
- *Adjustment No. 3*
  A physical inventory count indicates that $50,000 worth of initial supplies have been used.
- *Adjustment No. 4*
  The equipment of Alpha Hospital has an estimated useful life of ten years and the cost is being allocated over this time period. On a monthly basis this amounts to an allocation of $833 per month.
- *Adjustment No. 5*
  The building has an estimated useful life of forty years and the cost of this building is being allocated equally over its estimated life. On a monthly basis, this amounts to $4,167.
- *Adjustment No. 6*
  While no payment has occurred on either Notes Payable or Bonds Payable, it must be recognized that there is an interest expense associated with using money for this one month time period. This interest expense will be paid at a later date. Assume that the note payable carries an interest rate of 8% and the bond payable carries an interest rate of 6%. The actual amount of interest expense incurred for the month of January would be $8,167 ($667 on the note and $7,500 on the bond payable).

The effects of these adjustments on the balance sheet of Alpha Hospital, and on the ending balance sheet that would be prepared after all the adjustments were made are presented below.

Adjustment	Amount of Change	Account(s) Increased	Account(s) Decreased
No. 1	$100,000	Fund Balance	none
		Accounts Receivable	none
No. 2	50,000	Wages & Salaries Payable	Fund Balance
No. 3	50,000	none	Fund Balance Supplies
No. 4	833	none	Fund Balance, Equipment
No. 5	4,167	none	Fund Balance Building
No. 6	8,167	Interest Payable	Fund Balance

ALPHA HOSPITAL BALANCE SHEET
January 31, 1978

Assets		Liabilities And Fund Balance	
Cash	$320,000	Wages & Salary Payable	$50,000
Accounts Receivable	120,000	Interest Payable	8,167
Supplies	150,000	Note Payable	100,000
Equipment	99,167	Bonds Payable	1,500,000
Building	1,995,833	Fund Balance	1,026,833
TOTAL	$2,685,000	TOTAL	$2,685,000

It is also possible to prepare the following statement of revenues and expenses.

ALPHA HOSPITAL
STATEMENT OF REVENUES AND EXPENSES
For Month Ended January 31, 1978

Revenues	$200,000
Less Expenses	
Wages and Salaries	$110,000
Supplies	50,000
Depreciation	5,000
Interest	8,167
TOTAL	$173,167
Excess of Revenues over Expenses	$26,833

Note that the difference between revenue and expense during the month of January was $26,833, the exact amount by which the fund balance of Alpha Hospital changed during the month. Alpha Hospital began the month with $1,000,000 in its fund balance account and ended with $1,026,833. This illustrates an important point in the reading of financial statements: *the individual financial statements are fundamentally related to one another.*

Stable Monetary Unit

The money measurement principle of accounting discussed earlier restricted accounting measures to money. In accounting in the United States, the unit of measure is the U.S. dollar. At the present time no adjustment to changes in the general purchasing power of that unit is required in financial reports; a 1962 dollar is assumed to be equal in value to a 1977 dollar. This permits arithmetic operations such as addition and subtraction. If this assumption were not made, adding the unadjusted historical cost values of assets inquired in different time periods would be inappropriate, like adding apples and oranges. Current, generally accepted accounting principles incorporate this *stable monetary unit principle.*

This may not seem like a very major problem. In fact, when the inflation rate was less than two per cent annually, it really was not. However, in light of present rates of inflation, the effects of assuming a stable monetary unit can be quite dramatic. Imagine that the inflation rate in the economy is currently 100% compounded monthly. The hypothetical entity under consideration is a neighborhood health center that has all of its expenses, except payroll, covered by grants from governmental agencies. Its employees have a contract that automatically adjusts their wages to changes in the general price level. (With a monthly inflation rate of 100%, it is no wonder.) Assume that revenues from patients are collected on the first day of the month following the one in which they were billed, but that employees are paid at the beginning of each month. Rates to patients will be set so that the excess of revenues over expenses will be zero. With the first month's wages set equal to $100,000, the following Income and Cash Flow positions result for the first six months of the year:

	INCOME FLOWS			CASH FLOWS		
	Expense	Revenue	Net Income	Inflow	Outflow	Difference
January	$100,000	$100,000	0	$50,000*	$100,000	(50,000)
February	200,000	200,000	0	$100,000	200,000	(100,000)
March	400,000	400,000	0	200,000	400,000	(200,000)
April	800,000	800,000	0	400,000	800,000	(400,000)
May	1,600,000	1,600,000	0	800,000	1,600,000	(800,000)
June	3,200,000	3,200,000	0	1,600,000	3,200,000	(1,600,000)
	$6,300,000	$6,300,000	0	$3,150,000	$6,300,000	(3,150,000)

*$50,000 is equal to the revenue billed in December.

Note the tremendous difference between income and cash flow. While the income statement would indicate a break-even operation, the cash balance at the end of June would be a negative $3,150,000. Obviously, operations cannot continue indefinitely in light of the extreme cash hardship position imposed.

Fortunately, the rate of inflation in our economy is not 100%. However, smaller rates of inflation compounded over long periods of time could create similar problems. For example, limiting reimbursement of depreciation to an asset's unadjusted historical cost leaves the entity with a significant cash deficit when it is time to replace that asset. Yet, currently most third party payers do in fact limit reimbursement to unadjusted historical cost depreciation.

Fund Accounting

Fund accounting is a system in which an entity's assets and liabilities are segregated in the accounting records. Each fund may be thought of as an independent entity with its own self-balancing set of accounts. The basic accounting equation discussed under the duality principle must be satisfied for each fund—assets must equal liabilities plus fund balance for the particular fund in question. This is, in fact, how the term fund balance developed; a fund balance originally represented the residual interest for a *particular fund.*

Fund accounting is widely employed by nonprofit, voluntary health care facilities, especially hospitals. It is not a basic concept or principle of accounting like those previously discussed, but it is a feature peculiar to accounting for many health care organizations. It evolved primarily for use in stewarding funds donated by external parties where stipulations on the usage of those monies were imposed.

Two major categories of funds are presently used in the hospital industry and for other health care facilities. They are *restricted* and *unrestricted.* A restricted fund is one in which a third party, outside the entity, has imposed certain restrictions on use of donated monies or resources. There are three common types of restricted funds:

- Specific Purpose Funds
- Plant Replacement and Expansion Funds
- Endowment Funds

Specific purpose funds are donated by individuals or organizations and restricted for purposes other than plant replacement and expansion or endowment. Monies received from government agencies to perform specific research or other work are examples of specific purpose funds.

Plant replacement and expansion funds are restricted for use in plant replacement and expansion. Assets purchased with these monies are not recorded in this fund. When the monies are used for plant purposes, the amounts are transferred to the unrestricted fund. For example, if $200,000 in cash from the Plant Replacement Fund were used to acquire a piece of equipment, the equipment and fund balance of the Unrestricted Fund would be increased.

Endowment funds are contributed to be held intact for generating income. The income may or may not be restricted for specific purposes. Some endowments are classified as "term" endowments. That is, after the expiration of some time period, the restriction on use of the principal is lifted. The balance is then transferred to the unrestricted fund.

Unrestricted funds have no third party restrictions imposed upon them. In some cases, the governing board of the organization may restrict use, but since this is not an external or third party restriction, the funds are still classified as unrestricted. Sometimes the unrestricted fund is referred to as the general or operating fund.

CONVENTIONS OF ACCOUNTING

The accounting principles discussed up to this point are important in the preparation of financial statements. Several widely accepted conventions modify the application of these principles in certain circumstances. We shall discuss three of the more important ones:

- Conservatism
- Materiality
- Consistency

Conservatism affects the valuation of some assets. Specifically, accountants use a "lower of cost or market rule" for valuing inventories and marketable securities. The "lower of cost or market" rule means that the value of a stock of inventory or marketable securities would be its actual cost or market value, whichever is less. For these resources, there is a deviation from cost valuation to market valuation, whenever market value is lower.

Materiality permits certain transactions to be treated out of accordance with generally accepted accounting principles. This might be permitted because it does not materially affect the presentation of financial position. For example, theoretically paper clips have an estimated useful life greater than one year. However, the cost of capitalizing this item and systematically and rationally allocating it over its useful life is not justifiable; the difference in financial position that would be created by not using generally accepted accounting principles would be immaterial.

Consistency limits the accounting alternatives that can be used. In any given transaction, there is usually a variety of available, generally acceptable accounting treatments. For example, generally accepted accounting principles permit the use of double declining balance, sum of the year digits, or straight line methods for allocating the costs of depreciable assets over their estimated useful life, but the consistency convention limits an. entity's ability to change from one acceptable method to another. Recall that the opinion paragraph in a CPA's audit report assures that generally accepted accounting principles have been applied on a basis *consistent* with that of the previous year.

SUMMARY

In this chapter we have discussed the importance of generally accepted accounting principles in deriving financial information: though these principles are formally required only in the preparation of audited financial statements, they influence the derivation of most financial information. Understanding some of the basic principles is critical to understanding financial information in general.

Six specific principles of accounting were discussed in some detail:

- Accounting Entity
- Money Measurement
- Duality
- Cost Valuation
- Accrual Accounting
- Stable Monetary Unit

In addition to these, the general importance of fund accounting, as it relates to the hospital and health care industry, was also discussed. The chapter concluded with a discussion of three conventions which may modify the application of generally accepted accounting principles in specific situations.

With this basic groundwork, we will now examine the four financial statements which are the primary outputs of financial accounting.

Chapter 3

Financial Statements

Understanding the principles of accounting is a critical first step in understanding financial statements. However, the format and language of financial statements may be unintelligible to the occasional reader. This chapter will discuss in some detail the four major, general purpose financial statements:

- Balance Sheet—Exhibits 3-1 and 3-2
- Statement of Revenues and Expenses—Exhibit 3-3
- Statement of Changes in Financial Position—Exhibit 3-4
- Statement of Changes in Fund Balances—Exhibit 3-5

The balance sheet and statement of revenues and expenses are more widely published and used than the other two statements. Understanding them enables a reader to use the other two financial statements, and financial information in general. This chapter will pay major attention to the balance sheet and statement of revenue and expenses.

BALANCE SHEET (UNRESTRICTED FUNDS)

Examination of the balance sheets presented in Exhibits 3-1 and 3-2 illustrates the separation of funds into restricted and unrestricted categories. Restricted funds are not available for general operating purposes (Exhibit 3-2). The duality principle can also be seen operating in these balance sheets. Assets do equal liabilities plus fund balance, in both restricted and unrestricted balance sheets. Finally, the entity being accounted for is Omega Hospital.

27

Current Assets

Assets which are expected to be exchanged for cash or consumed during the operating cycle of the entity (or one year, if longer) are classified as current assets on the balance sheet. The operating cycle is the length of time between acquisition of materials and services and collection of revenue generated by them. Since the operating cycle for most health care organizations is significantly less than one year (perhaps three months or less), current assets are predominantly those which may be expected to be converted into cash or used to reduce expenditures of cash within one year.

Cash

Cash represents the funds on hand in bill or coin form or in savings or checking accounts. It does not include funds restricted in some way, for example, cash funds restricted for investment in retirement plans or self-insurance plans.

Marketable Securities

Marketable securities, or short-term investments, comprise another major category of current assets that often shows up on balance sheets, although it is not shown in Exhibit 3-1. In some cases, cash and marketable securities will be combined. This is not considered bad reporting because the liquidity of marketable securities allows them to be treated as cash for most purposes. Marketable securities are short-term investments that meet two criteria. First, management must intend to sell or convert them to cash within a year's time. This is guaranteed if the maturity of the investment is less than one year. Second, they must have a readily available and active market. Marketable securities are valued at their cost or market value, whichever is lower. This is one of the few exceptions to the cost valuation principle.

Accounts Receivable

Accounts receivable represent legally enforceable claims on customers for prior services or goods. In Omega Hospital, there are two categories of accounts receivable: patient and other. Other accounts receivable in a health care organization imply revenue derived from sources other than patient services. For example, Omega Hospital has a physician's office building, a parking ramp and a number of educational programs. Accounts receivable may exist in one or all of those areas.

Patient accounts receivable are usually the largest accounts receivable item, and for that matter, the largest single current asset item in the balance sheet. Omega Hospital is no exception—it has an estimated $3,675,531 in accounts receivable that will eventually result in cash. The actual dollar amount of accounts receivable is higher, but is reduced by estimated allowances.

A characteristic of hospitals and other health care organizations which makes their accounts receivable different from most other organization's is that charges actually billed to patients are quite often settled for substantially less than amounts charged. The differences are also known as allowances. Four major categories of allowances are used to restate accounts receivable to expected, realizable value:

- Charity Allowances
- Courtesy Allowances
- Doubtful Account Allowances
- Contractual Allowances

A charity allowance is the difference between established service rates and amounts actually charged to indigent patients. Many health care facilities have a policy of scaling the normal charge by some factor based on income, especially in clinics and other ambulatory care settings. A courtesy allowance is the difference between established rates for services and rates billed special patients, such as employees, doctors and clergy. A doubtful account allowance is the difference between rates billed and amounts expected to be recovered. For example, a medically indigent patient might actually receive services that have an established rate of $100, but be billed only $50. If it is anticipated that the patient will not pay even the $50, then that $50 will show up as a doubtful account allowance.

A contractual allowance may be the largest of accounts receivable deductions in many situations. It falls in a deduction category that may be new to many readers of financial statements. A contractual allowance is the difference between rates billed patients for services and the amounts to be paid by their third party payers. Many third party payers, Medicare, Medicaid, and Blue Cross, have contractual relations with the health care facility that limit payment to costs as defined in some prescribed manner. Cost based reimbursement is usually less than charges. In other situations a third party payer, such as Blue Cross or Medicaid, may limit payment specifying that it will pay a certain percentage of billed charges.

It is important to note that the allowances are estimates and will, in all probability, differ from the actual value of accounts receivable eventually written off. For example, Omega Hospital shows an expected value of accounts receivable to be collected of $3,675,531 in 1976, but actually has $4,283,531 of outstanding accounts receivable.

$3,675,531	Net Accounts Receivable
278,000	Contractual Allowances
330,000	Doubtful Account Allowance
$4,283,531	Accounts Receivable Gross

Since estimation of allowances is so critical to the reported value of accounts receivable, the methodology should be scrutinized. Just how was the estimate developed? Has the estimating method been used in the past with any degree of reliability? An external audit performed by an independent CPA can usually provide this degree of reliability and assurance.

Inventories

Inventories in a health care facility represent items that are to be used in the delivery of health care services. They may range from normal business office supplies to highly specialized chemicals used in a laboratory.

Prepaid Expenses

Prepaid expenses represent expenditures already made for future service. In Omega Hospital they may represent prepayment of insurance premiums for the year, rents on leased equipment or other items. For example, an insurance premium for a professional liability insurance policy may be $600,000 per year, due one year in advance. If this amount were paid on January 1st, then on June 30th, $300,000, or one-half the total, would be shown as a prepaid expense.

Property and Equipment

This category is sometimes called Fixed Assets or shown more descriptively as Plant Property and Equipment. Items in this category represent investment in tangible, permanent assets, and are sometimes referred to as the capital assets of the organization. These items are shown at the historical cost or acquisition cost, reduced by allowances for depreciation.

Land and Improvements

Land and improvements represent the historical cost of the earth's surface owned by the health care facility and the historical cost of any improvements erected on it. Such improvements might be water and sewer systems, roadways, fences, sidewalks, shrubbery and parking lots. While land may not be depreciated, land improvements may. Land held for investment purposes will not be shown in this category, but will appear as an investment in the other assets section.

Buildings and Equipment

Buildings and equipment represent all buildings and equipment owned by the entity and used in the normal course of its operations. These items are also stated at the historical cost. Buildings and equipment not used in the normal course of operations should be reported separately. For example, real estate investments would not be shown in the fixed asset or plant property and equipment section, but in the other assets section. Equipment in many situations is classified into three categories: (1) *fixed equipment*—affixed to the building in which it is located, including items such as elevators, boilers and generators; (2) *major movable equipment*—usually stationary but capable of being moved, including reasonably expensive items such as automobiles, laboratory equipment and x-ray apparatus; and (3) *minor equipment*—usually low in cost with short estimated useful lives, including such items as wastebaskets, glassware and sheets.

Construction in Progress

Construction in progress represents the amount of money that has been expended on projects which are still not complete at the date the financial statement is published. In Omega Hospital there are currently $25,741,801 of building additions in progress and $377,317 of other construction in progress. When these projects are *completed*, the values will be charged to buildings and equipment.

Allowance for Depreciation

Allowance for depreciation represents the accumulated depreciation taken on the asset to date of the financial statement. The concept of depreciation is important and useful in a wide number of decisions. The following example illustrates the depreciation concept.

A $500 desk is purchased and depreciated over a five-year life. Balance sheet values are presented below.

	Year				
	1	2	3	4	5
Historical Equipment Cost	$500	$500	$500	$500	$500
Allowance for Depreciation	100	200	300	400	500
Net	$400	$300	$200	$100	$ 0

In the case of Omega Hospital, there is $6,745,307 of accumulated depreciation at June 30, 1976. The historical cost base for this amount is probably fairly close to $11,191,834, the historical cost value of buildings and equipment. In reality, the figure is slightly higher because land improvements are also depreciated and would be included in the accumulated depreciation total. This means that 60.26% of the historical cost of present facilities has been depreciated in prior years. As the ratio of allowance for depreciation to building and equipment increases, it usually signifies that a physical plant will need replacement in the near future. Omega Hospital appears to be in such a situation, which may partially explain the current construction.

Other Assets

Other assets are assets that are neither current nor involve plant and equipment. Typically they are either investments or intangible assets. In the case of Omega Hospital, all other assets consist of investments that have been Board restricted; they must be shown in the unrestricted balance sheet because the Board restriction does not qualify as a third party restriction. However, they are shown separately in the unrestricted balance sheet to identify the restriction.

Two major intangible asset items that show up in some health care facility balance sheets are Goodwill and Organization Costs. Goodwill represents the difference between the price paid to acquire another entity, and the fair market value of the acquired entity's assets less any related obligations or liabilities. Goodwill shows up mainly in proprietary facilities. Organization costs are expended for legal and accounting fees and other items incurred at the formation of an entity. The cost of these items is usually amortized over some allowable life.

Current Liabilities

Current liabilities are obligations which are expected to require payment in cash during the coming year or operating cycle, whichever is longer. Like current assets, they are generally expected to be paid in one year's time.

Accounts Payable

Accounts payable may be thought of as the counterpart of accounts receivable. They represent the entity's promise to pay money for goods or services it has received. In the Omega Hospital example, two types of accounts payable appear, one resulting from normal activity, called Accounts Payable-Trade, the other due to the construction contractor for work in process, referred to as Accounts Payable-Construction Contractor.

Advances from Third Parties

Advances from third parties comprise an account that is somewhat peculiar to the health care industry. In some situations a third party payer, Blue Cross particularly, will pay a health care entity a sum in advance of the provision of services. Since the entity must generally invest its resources prior to payment, this advance partially offsets the entity's requirement for a cash outflow and helps meet the financial requirements of the health care facility. An additional advantage is that the advance may reduce the amount of money a health care provider must borrow; this reduces interest expense and thereby keeps costs down in the long run.

Accrued Expenses

Accrued expenses are obligations that result from prior operations. They are thus a present right or enforceable demand. For example, in Chapter 2 the accruing of interest expense with the passage of time was discussed. Some other examples of accrued expenses would be payroll, vacation pay, tax deductions, rent and insurance. In some cases accrued expenses are disaggregated to show material categories, especially payroll. Omega Hospital does not do this, but does show a separate listing of payroll deductions.

Payroll Deductions

Payroll deductions represent amounts withheld from the employees' wages to meet a variety of federal, state and local obligations for example social security contributions and income taxes.

Current Maturities of Long-Term Debt

Current maturities of long-term debt represent the amount of *principal* that will be repaid on the indebtedness within the coming year. It does not equal the total amount of the payments that will be made during that year. Total payments will include both interest and principal, current maturities of long term debt include just the principal portion. For example, if at the June 30th fiscal year close, a total of $360,000 ($30,000 per month) will be paid on long term indebtedness during the coming year, and of this amount only $120,000 is principal payment, then $120,000 would be shown as a current maturity of long term debt.

Noncurrent Liabilities

Noncurrent liabilities include obligations that will not require payment in cash for at least one year or more. Omega Hospital shows two types of noncurrent liabilities. Mortgage Payable and Loan Payable from Restricted Fund.

Mortgage Payable

Mortgage payable is one source of long-term indebtedness. The adjective mortgage implies that the indebtedness is collateralized by a lien on some set of the entity's assets. Other examples of long-term debt are bonds payable and notes payable.

Loan Payable (Restricted Fund)

Omega Hospital also has a noncurrent liability described as loan payable from restricted funds. This brings up an important issue. Just how valid is this liability? The debt is, after all, owed to the entity itself. Note that at June 30, 1975, the indebtedness of $554,689 is classified as a current liability, but on June 30, 1976 the indebtedness of $1,390,905 is classified as noncurrent. This transfer from current liabilities to noncurrent liabilities causes some speculation about the validity of the indebtedness. However, it must be remembered that a restricted fund is one in which a third party has imposed some restrictions on use. The validity of the loan, as well as the separation of funds, depends upon the legitimacy of those restrictions.

Deferred Revenue

Deferred revenue is not classified as liability or fund balance. Deferred revenue means cash or other assets received prior to the actual recognition of the amount as revenue. Typically, in the health care industry, the deferred revenue account is used to recognize timing differences between the receipt of cash and the recognition as revenue. For example, Omega Hospital may have used some form of accelerated depreciation for cost reimbursement purposes, but used straight line depreciation for financial reporting. Specifically, in the desk illustration discussed earlier, straight line depreciation in the first year would be $100. If the *sum of the year's digits* depreciation method were used for reimbursement purposes, first year depreciation would be $167. The difference ($67) would be recorded as deferred revenue. At the conclusion of the useful life of this asset, the deferred revenue account would be "0".

Fund Balance

Fund balance, as discussed earlier, represents the difference between assets and the claim to those assets by third parties or liabilities. Increases in this account balance usually arise from one of two sources:

- Contributions
- Earnings

In the nonprofit health care industry, there is usually no separation in the fund balance account recognizing these two sources. Thus, there is no indication of how much of Omega Hospital's fund balance of $8,813,024 was earned and how much was contributed. Financial statements prepared for proprietary entities do show this break down. Earnings of prior years, reduced by dividend payments to stockholders, are shown in an account labeled Retained Earnings.

In any given year, however, it is possible to determine the sources of change in fund balance by examining the Statement of Changes in Fund Balance (Exhibit 3-5). For example, in fiscal year 1976 transfers from the plant replacement and renovation fund, a restricted fund, accounted for all the increase in fund balance. These transfers more than offset the operating loss of $226,247 for the period.

The value of the fund balance account at any point in time is often confused with the cash position of the entity. Cash and fund balance will hardly ever be equal. In most situations, the cash balance will be far less than fund balance. For example, Omega Hospital has $8,812,307 in fund balance at June 30, 1976, but only $376,766 in cash at the same date. Assuming that the $8,812,307 reported as fund balance can be converted into cash is a false assumption.

BALANCE SHEET (RESTRICTED FUNDS)

The balance sheet of Omega Hospital has a separate accounting for four funds which third parties have restricted:

- Special Purpose Fund
- Research Fund
- Endowment Fund
- Plant Replacement and Renovation Fund

It is possible to think of these four funds as separate balance sheets each satisfying the basic accounting equation of

$$assets = liabilities + fund\ balance.$$

For example, the plant replacement and renovation fund has a fund balance of $3,378,408 which must equal its assets because no liabilities exist. The assets of the plant replacement and renovation fund consist of $1,681,258 in cash and money market investments, $306,245 in pledges receivable, and $1,390,905 in loans receivable from unrestricted funds.

OMEGA HOSPITAL
BALANCE SHEET
Plant Replacement and Renovation Fund

Assets		Fund Balance	
Cash & Money Market Investments	$1,681,258	Fund Balance	$3,378,408
Pledges Receivable	306,245		$3,378,408
Loan Receivable-Unrestricted Fund	1,390,905		
TOTAL	$3,378,408		

This arithmetic is also representative for the other three funds.

The use of the cost valuation principle can be seen clearly in the investments of the endowment fund. In 1975 and 1976, the market value of the investments was less than their historical cost, but cost valuation continued to be used. In reality, Omega Hospital does not have $685,815 in endowment fund investments, but only a realizable value of $575,431. This difference could be caused by poor investment management or external limitations on investment, imposed by the stipulations of the initial gift. Regardless of the reason, the hospital has seen a decline in its initial, donated value of $110,384. (See Exhibit 3-2.)

Pledges receivable is an account that may be unfamiliar to many individuals. It represents a legally enforceable commitment from a third party. In the case of Omega Hospital, $306,245 of pledges are currently outstanding as of June 30, 1976. These pledges are restricted and must be used for plant replacement and renovation. Restricted in this way, they will never be have to be reported as income by Omega Hospital. Depending upon management's objectives, it may or it may not be advantageous to restrict the majority of gifts. For example, a hospital faced with regulatory controls on income may wish to restrict all pledges so it will not have to report them as income. Nonetheless, it is important to recognize such sources of unreported income in the assessment of a health care entity's financial strength.

STATEMENT OF REVENUE AND EXPENSE

The Statement of Revenue and Expense has become a financial statement of increasing importance, both in the proprietary and nonproprietary sector. It gives more individuals a better picture of operations in a given time period than a balance sheet does. A balance sheet summarizes the wealth position of an entity at a given point in time by delineating its assets, liabilities and fund balance. An income statement provides information concerning *how* that wealth position was changed through operations.

An entity's ability to earn an excess of revenue over expenses is an important variable in many external and internal decisions. A series of income statements indicates this ability well. Creditors use income statements to determine the entity's ability to pay future and present debts; management and rate regulating agencies use them to assess whether current and proposed rate structures are adequate.

The *entity* principle is an important factor in analyzing and interpreting the statement of revenue and expense. Income—the excess of revenue over expenses comes from a large number of individual operations within a health care entity—is *aggregated* in the statement of revenue and expense. Minor breakdowns, for example, on a departmental basis may be required for some decisions: little can be said about specific rates and their adequacy within a health care facility if departmental statements of revenue and expense are not available. These statements *are* frequently available and should be used. However, this chapter will focus on the general purpose statement of revenue and expense which is an aggregate of the individual departments' income.

Revenue

Generally, speaking, revenue in a health care facility comes from three sources:

1. operations related to patient services
2. operations not related to patient services
3. nonoperating sources

Patient Service Revenue

Patient service revenue in most facilities is by far the largest source of revenue. Omega Hospital reported $23,448,220 of patient service revenue in 1976. This amount is stated at its gross or billed value and does not reflect what amounts were actually collected or expected to be collected. To determine what was or will be collected, the gross figure must be reduced by estimates of the four categories of allowances discussed earlier in the chapter. Omega Hospital had $1,208,376 of allowances and uncollectible accounts in 1976 which yielded a net patient services revenue of $22,239,844. Net patient service revenue reflects the amount of revenue that will be realized in cash payments; it measures what is or will be collected, not what was charged.

Earlier discussion of accounts receivable briefly mentioned the four categories of allowances (charity, courtesy, contractual and uncollectible) that must be estimated to state accounts receivable properly in terms of realizable cash value. Note that the value of the estimated allowances for accounts receivable in 1976 (Exhibit 3-1) is

$$278,000 + \$330,000 = \$608,000.$$

This figure is significantly less than the amount shown in the statement of revenue and expenses for allowances, $1,208,376. This relationship is quite common. Remember that the balance sheet value reflects the estimated allowances for accounts still outstanding, but the statement of revenue and expenses value reflects the allowance for all patient service revenue billed during the year.

Certain categories of patient service revenue are important in decision making. Payment source is especially important. Some common categories of payment sources are—

- Medicare
- Medicaid
- Blue Cross

- Commercial Insurance
- Self Pay
- Other

Identifying these categories is critical to setting rates and making many other financial decisions, such as projection of short-term cash flow and collection efforts. Ordinarily this information is available within the entity, though it is not usually published in general purpose financial statements. Departmental breakdowns are also useful in many decisions and available internally, but not usually published in general purpose financial statements.

Other Operating Revenue

Other operating revenue is generated from normal, day-to-day operations not directly related to patient care. It is usually classified by source into three categories: (1) educational programs, (2) grants, and (3) miscellaneous. Revenue from such educational programs as nursing, medicine, laboratory or x-ray technology may generate tuition and other fees which show up in this category. Omega Hospital has a relatively large dollar amount of other operating revenue—$665,160 in 1976—much of it represents tuition from educational programs.

Grants from research projects or projects run by federal or other agencies are also reported as other operating revenue. Omega Hospital has some monies in this category, shown in the statement of changes in fund balances (Exhibit 3-5). A transfer of $75,775 was made from the restricted research fund to the unrestricted fund as other operating revenue in 1976.

Miscellaneous sources of other operating revenue include such items as revenue from office rentals, cafeteria and gift shop sales, and parking lot fees. It is important to note that this revenue is not always offset against its related expenses. As a result, it is sometimes impossible to determine whether these operations were profitable or not. If they are immaterial, their value determination is not an important problem. On the contrary, Omega Hospital, for example, believes that its parking lot and professional office building operations are significant enough to warrant separate reporting. Therefore, in Omega's statement of revenue and expenses, this revenue is netted against related expenses, rather than appearing just as other operating revenue.

Nonoperating Revenue

Nonoperating revenue is revenue not related to patient care or to normal, day-to-day operations. Major categories of nonoperating revenue are: (1) unrestricted gifts, (2) unrestricted income from endowments, and (3) miscellaneous.

Unrestricted gifts—gifts with no restrictions on use—are treated as nonoperating revenue. Omega Hospital had relatively few of these gifts in the two years of reports for which we have information. However, Omega Hospital did receive a large dollar amount of gifts restricted for plant replacement and renovation in the past, as evidenced by the values for pledges receivable shown in the restricted balance sheet.

If income from an endowment is not restricted, it may be used for general operating purposes and treated as nonoperating revenue. The statement of changes in fund balances (Exhibit 3-5) shows that only $2,018 of income was designated as nonoperating revenue in 1976.

Miscellaneous sources include income from unrestricted funds, rentals of facilities not used in operations, such as farm land or apartments, and in some cases the fair market value of services donated by volunteers.

Operating Expenses

In these days of increasing concern over health care costs, many decision makers are paying more attention to health care facilities' operating expenses. Generally speaking, there are two ways that expenses may be categorized: (1) by cost or responsibility center, and (2) by object or type of expenditure.

In most general purpose financial statements, costs are reported by cost center or department. Omega Hospital breaks down expenses into five major categories of departments:

- Nursing service areas
- Other professional service areas
- General service areas
- Fiscal service areas
- Administrative service areas

Nursing service and other professional services could also be classified as revenue departments. They provide services directly to patients for which there is a charge. General, fiscal and administrative services are indirect or support areas. They do not provide direct patient services, but support the nursing and other professional service areas.

Two expenses, depreciation and interest, are listed by object or type of expense category. As we will see in the next chapter, these two expense categories are critical to many decisions and require separate reporting.

It should be noted that expense and expenditure (or payment oi cash) may not be equivalent in any given period. For example, a health care facility may incur an expenditure of $1,000,000 to buy a piece of equipment, but may only charge $200,000 as depreciation expense in a given year. In general, expenditure reflects the payment of cash, while expense recognizes prior expenditure that has produced revenue. In general, there are three major categories of expenditures that are not treated as expenses:

1. retirement or repayment of debt
2. investment in new fixed assets
3. increases in working capital or current assets

One major category of expense, depreciation on fixed assets, does not involve a cash expenditure.

STATEMENT OF CHANGES IN FINANCIAL POSITION

The Statement of Changes in Financial Position is designed to give more information on the flow of funds within an entity. As we just discussed, the concept of expense does not necessarily give decision makers information on funds flow. The Statement of Changes in Financial Position is designed to give more information on the flow of funds within an entity—to summarize the sources which make funds available and the uses for those funds during a given period.

Funds are usually defined as working capital. This is true for Omega Hospital in Exhibit 3-4. Major categories of fund sources include—

- income-related sources
- debt financing
- sale of assets

Major uses of funds include—

- purchase of fixed assets
- repayment of debt
- increases in working capital

Income-related sources consist of the difference between revenue and expenses, plus the related depreciation expense. Depreciation is added back to income because depreciation does not involve an actual expenditure of cash or funds. Many financial analysts refer to the sum of depreciation and net income as cash flow. In Omega Hospital, net operating income before depreciation was $500,345 which equals $549,799 of depreciation less the $49,454 operating loss (Exhibit 3-4).

STATEMENT OF CHANGES IN FUND BALANCE

The Statement of Changes in Fund Balance for both unrestricted and restricted funds merely accounts for the changes in fund balance during the year. Information on flow between restricted and unrestricted fund, and flows into the entity that are restricted, can be identified from this statement.

In fiscal years 1975 and 1976, Omega Hospital has had a lot of activity in the Plant Replacement and Renovation Fund. The fund has received $363,000 in Hill-Burton construction grants, earned $412,530 in interest on its investment and received $174,383 in pledges. Such transactions are never reported as income in a statement of revenues and expenses, but they did have a very positive effect on the Omega Hospital's financial position. Close scrutiny of the statement of changes in fund balance can detect many of these flows.

SUMMARY

In this chapter we have discussed the contents of four general purpose financial statements:

- Balance Sheet
- Statement of Revenues and Expenses
- Statement of Changes in Financial Position
- Statement of Changes in Fund Balances

Primary attention was directed at the first two, Balance Sheet and Statement of Revenues and Expenses, which provide a basis for most financial information.

Our attention in this chapter was directed at understanding the basic information available in these four financial statements. The next two chapters will discuss how that information can be interpreted and used in actual decision making.

Exhibit 3-1

Omega Hospital
Balance Sheet
Unrestricted Funds
June 30, 1976

(with comparative figures for 1975)

ASSETS	June 30 1976	June 30 1975
CURRENT		
Cash	$ 376,766	$ 46,073
Accounts receivable		
Patients (less contractual allowances from third party payers of $278,000 in 1976 and $248,000 in 1975, and allowance for doubtful accounts of $330,000 in 1976 and $295,000 in 1975)	3,675,531	2,846,266
Other	272,144	260,070
Inventories	325,720	255,176
Prepaid expenses	343,640	289,806
TOTAL CURRENT ASSETS	4,993,801	3,697,391
PROPERTY AND EQUIPMENT		
Land and improvements	413,809	408,557
Buildings and equipment	11,191,834	10,776,959
Building additions in progress	25,741,801	18,199,040
Other construction in progress	377,317	36,502
	37,724,761	29,421,058
Allowances for depreciation	6,745,307	6,106,815
TOTAL PROPERTY & EQUIPMENT	30,979,454	23,314,243

Exhibit 3-1 continued

OTHER

Board designated investments	98,328	102,470
	$36,071,583	$27,114,104

LIABILITIES, RESERVE AND FUND BALANCE	June 30 1976	June 30 1975
CURRENT LIABILITIES		
Accounts payable-trade	$ 797,966	$ 760,920
-construction contractor	1,665,797	1,724,878
Advances from third party payers	142,051	—
Loan payable-restricted Fund	—	554,689
Accrued expenses	1,341,393	868,091
Payroll deductions	127,478	143,017
Current maturities or mortgages payable	222,386	—
TOTAL CURRENT LIABILITIES	4,297,071	4,051,595
MORTGAGES PAYABLE	21,515,300	14,440,202
LOAN PAYABLE-RESTRICTED FUND	1,390,905	—
TOTAL LIABILITIES	27,203,276	18,491,797
DEFERRED REVENUE	56,000	76,000
FUND BALANCE	8,812,307	8,546,307
TOTAL	$36,071,583	$27,114,104

Exhibit 3-2

Omega Hospital
Balance Sheet
Restricted Funds
June 30, 1976

(with comparative figures for 1975)

	June 30	
ASSETS	1976	1975
Cash and money market investments		
Specific purpose funds	$ 117,889	$ 92,156
Research funds	57,848	46,347
Endowment funds	62,161	52,096
Plant replacement and renovation fund	1,681,258	2,248,863
Investments-Endowment Funds, at cost (approximate market value $575,431 in 1976 and $538,000 in 1975)	685,815	685,815
Plant replacement and renovation fund		
Pledges receivable	306,245	678,662
Loan receivable from unrestricted fund	1,390,905	554,689
	$4,302,121	$4,358,628
FUND BALANCE		
Specific purpose funds	$ 117,889	$ 92,156
Research funds	57,848	46,347
Endowment funds		
Free care	598,426	598,426
Scholarships	111,529	112,212
Other	38,021	27,273
Plant replacement and renovation fund	3,378,408	3,482,214
	$4,302,121	$4,358,628

Exhibit 3-3

Omega Hospital
Statement of Revenues and Expenses
Year Ended June 30, 1976
(with comparative figures for 1975)

	Year Ended June 30	
	1976	1975
HOSPITAL SERVICES		
Patient service revenue	$23,448,220	$19,814,924
Allowances and uncollectible accounts	1,208,376	751,475
Patient service revenue, before contractual allowances	22,239,844	19,063,449
Other operating revenue	665,160	614,834
TOTAL OPERATING REVENUE	22,905,004	19,678,283
OPERATING EXPENSES		
Nursing services	7,331,032	6,329,254
Other professional services	7,273,611	6,303,910
General services	3,769,307	3,086,584
Fiscal services	1,002,768	869,857
Administrative services	2,871,246	1,902,813
Provision for depreciation	549,799	470,609
Interest Expense	156,695	85,266
TOTAL OPERATING EXPENSES	22,954,458	19,048,293
Excess (deficiency) of operating revenues over operating expenses	(49,454)	629,990
NONOPERATING REVENUES	11,126	67,989
Excess (deficiency) of revenues over expenses	(38,328)	697,979

PROFESSIONAL OFFICE
  BUILDING SERVICES

    Excess of expenses over revenues   (80,420)   —

PARKING RAMP SERVICE

    Excess of expenses over revenues   (107,499)   —

EXCESS (DEFICIENCY) OF
  REVENUES OVER EXPENSES $(226,247) $ 697,979

Exhibit 3-4

Omega Hospital
Statement of Changes in Financial Position,
Unrestricted Funds,
Year Ended June 30, 1976

	12 Months to June 30, 1976
SOURCE OF FUNDS	
Net operating income before depreciation	$ 500,345
Nonoperating income	11,126
Professional office building income before depreciation	(2,883)
Parking Ramp income before depreciation	31,253
Loan from restricted funds	1,390,905
Increase in mortgage payable	7,075,098
Hill-Burton construction grant	128,000
Decrease in other assets	4,142
Transferred from restricted fund for plant renovation and equipment	364,247
TOTAL SOURCES OF FUNDS	$9,502,233
USES OF FUNDS	
Purchase of fixed assets	888,538
Construction of new facilities	7,542,761
Decrease in deferred revenue	20,000
Increase in working capital	1,050,934
TOTAL USES OF FUND	$9,502,233
CHANGES IN WORKING CAPITAL	
Increase in current assets	$1,296,410
Less increase in current liabilities	245,476
INCREASE IN WORKING CAPITAL	$1,050,934

Exhibit 3-5

Omega Hospital Statement of Changes in Fund Balances,
Year Ended June 30, 1976 (with comparative figures for 1975)

	Year Ended June 30	
	1976	1975
UNRESTRICTED FUNDS		
Balance at beginning of year	$8,546,307	$7,129,625
Excess (deficiency) of revenues over expenses	(226,247)	697,979
Transfers from plant replacement and renovation fund to purchase property and equipment		
Hill-Burton construction grant	128,000	235,000
Renovation construction	302,032	450,110
Other donations and bequests	62,215	33,593
BALANCE AT END OF YEAR	$8,812,307	$8,546,307
RESTRICTED FUNDS		
Specific purpose funds		
Balance at beginning of year	$ 92,156	$ 83,586
Increases		
Contributions	40,019	30,472
Grants	28,397	10,478
Nursing school tuition & fees	57,851	47,312
Nursing student loan repayments	4,585	5,404
Transfer from endowment funds	3,781	3,912
TOTAL INCREASES	134,633	97,578
Decreases		
Specific purpose disbursements	24,512	19,482
Transfers to unrestricted fund		
Operating revenue or expense	51,037	42,085
Nursing student scholarships	13,148	12,116

Exhibit 3-5 continued

	Year Ended June 30	
Decreases (continued)	1976	1975
Property and equipment	14,134	—
Transfer to plant replacement and renovation fund	—	8,079
Student loan cancellation and repayment of government student loan advances and contra-adjustments	6,069	7,246
	108,900	89,008
BALANCE AT END OF YEAR	$ 117,889	$ 92,156

RESEARCH FUNDS

Balance at beginning of year	$ 46,347	$ 44,942
Increases		
Contributions and bequests	3,688	1,584
Grants	83,588	151,208
TOTAL INCREASES	87,276	152,792
Decreases		
Transfers to unrestricted funds (operating revenues)	75,775	151,387
Balance at end of year	$ 57,848	$ 46,347

ENDOWMENT FUNDS

Balance at beginning of year	$ 737,911	$ 741,133
Increases		
Income from investments	43,898	49,430

Exhibit 3-5 continued

Decreases	Year Ended June 30	
	1976	1975
Transfers to unrestricted funds		
Operating revenue	22,311	36,497
Non-operating revenue	2,018	2,022
Endowment fund disbursements	5,723	10,221
Transfers to specific purpose funds	3,781	3,912
TOTAL DECREASES	33,833	52,652
Balance at end of year	$ 747,976	$ 737,911

Plant replacement and renovation fund

	1976	1975
Balance at beginning of year	$3,482,214	$3,539,497
Increases		
Contributions	2,125	2,015
Hill-Burton construction grant	128,000	235,000
Interest earned	187,667	224,863
Donated equipment	62,215	25,514
Transfer from specific purpose funds	—	8,079
Pledges receivable from building fund campaign	8,434	165,949
TOTAL INCREASES	388,441	661,420
Decreases		
Transfers to unrestricted fund		
Hill-Burton construction grant	128,000	235,000
Renovation construction	302,032	450,110
Donated property and equipment	62,215	33,593
TOTAL DECREASES	492,247	718,703
Balance at end of year	$3,378,408	$3,482,214

Chapter 4

Analyzing Financial Statements

The major purpose of this chapter is to introduce some analytic tools for evaluating the financial condition of health care entities. Think for a moment how confusing and difficult it would be to reach any decisions on Omega Hospital's financial condition as it is presented in Exhibits 3-1, 3-2, 3-3, 3-4 and 3-5, without a key. Unless your training is in business or finance, the statements may look like a mass of endless numbers with little meaning. In short, there may be too much information in most financial statements to be digested easily by a general purpose user.

An exhaustive list of people who might use general purpose financial information would be difficult to prepare. Some of the potential users and their purposes for measuring financial condition are listed below:

1. Board of Trustees—to evaluate the solvency of their facility and establish a framework for various decisions such as investment, financing and pricing.

2. Health Systems Agencies—to review the financial feasibility of projects and the financial condition of the proposed facility as mandated in Section 1122 of the Social Security Act of 1972.

3. Creditors—to determine the amounts and terms of credit to be granted health care facilities and to evaluate the security of presently outstanding credit obligations.

4. Employee Unions—to evaluate the financial condition of a health care facility and its ability to meet increasing demands for higher wages; also to assess the capability of the facility to meet existing contractual relationships for deferred compensation programs such as pension plans.

5. Departmental Managers—to understand better how operations and activities under their direct control contribute to the entity's overall financial position.

6. Rate Regulation Agencies—to assess the adequacy of existing and proposed rates of a health care facility which is subject to rate review.

7. Grant Giving Agencies (Public and Private)—to determine a grantee's ability to continue to provide services supported by a grant and to assess the need for additional funding.

8. Public—to determine a community health care facility's financial condition and assess its need for rate increases and its use of prior funds to enhance and improve the delivery of health care services in order to assess the need for money in a fund drive.

RATIO ANALYSIS

The technique that will be used to assess financial condition is financial ratio analysis, the relation of two pieces of financial information to obtain additional information. In this process the new information is both easier to understand and usually more relevant than unrelated, freestanding information found in general purpose financial statements. For example, the values of fund balance and total assets may have little meaning when stated independently in a balance sheet. When the ratio of the two is taken, however, it indicates the proportion of assets that have been financed with sources other than debt.

Financial ratios are not another attempt by financial specialists to confuse and confound decision makers. Financial ratios have been empirically tested to determine their value in predicting business failure. The results to date have been quite impressive: financial ratios can discern potential problems in financial condition even five years in advance.

A sad fact is that much financial information is never really subjected to financial ratio analysis. As a result, the mass of figures just seems too voluminous ever to be synthesized: decision makers tend to assume that if the entity is breathing at the end of the year and is capable of publishing a financial statement, all must be well. If something goes wrong later, the accountant is blamed for not warning the decision makers. Sometimes the accountant *is* at fault. However, it is often the decision makers' fault for not analyzing and interpreting the financial information given to them in published financial statements.

The accounting profession was bombarded with criticism after the Penn Central collapse in 1970. To many it seemed that reporting standards must be too loose if an approximately seven-billion-dollar business could go under and its imminent financial collapse could not be determined from its financial statements. However Paul Dasher, in the March-April 1972 issue of the *Financial Analyst's Journal,* showed that anyone applying normal financial ratios to published financial statements could have detected the impending failure. At the conclusion of this chapter, you should be able to examine selectively a few specific financial ratios to better assess the financial condition of a health care entity.

Meaningful ratio analysis relies heavily upon the existence of relevant, comparable data. Absolute values of ratios are usually more valuable than the underlying financial information, but they are even more valuable when they can be compared to existing standards. For example, to say that a hospital earned three percent on its revenues in the previous year is useful, but to relate this three percent to some standard would be far more valuable.

Usually the analysis of financial ratios involves two types of comparisons. Temporal comparison of ratios, comparison of year-end ratios to prior year values, gives the analyst some idea of both trend and desirability. A projected financial ratio may similarly be compared to prior, actual values to test the validity of the projection and the desirability of the proposed plan of operation.

A second method of comparison uses industry averages as the relevant standards for comparison. The values for these standards are becoming more available as national and regional associations of health care organizations begin to assemble and periodically publish industry averages for selected ratios.

The lack of uniformity in financial reporting has inhibited meaningful financial analysis in the health care industry for some time. Specifically, the use of fund accounting has made it difficult to separate the financial effects of operations from the financial effects of other activities of the organization such as those supported by endowment or grant monies. To some extent this problem has been solved with the publication of the American Institute of Certified Public Accountants' *Hospital Audit Guide* in 1972. This publication, while technically applicable only for audited hospital financial statements, has affected financial reporting of other health care entities. Its major feature is the requirement that funds be separated into restricted and unrestricted categories, as discussed in the last chapter. In most situations, focussing the financial analysis on the unrestricted fund categories provides a better basis for evaluating actual health care operations.

Financial ratios will be classified into four major categories for the purposes of this chapter:

1. liquidity ratios
2. capital structure ratios
3. activity ratios
4. profitability ratios

Individual ratios within each of these categories will be defined and discussed with respect to their assessment of financial condition. The financial statements of Willkram Hospital, shown in Exhibits 4-1 and 4-2, will be used to illustrate the discussion.

It may seem that undue emphasis is being placed on financial reporting and financial analysis in the hospital sector. In terms of coverage in this chapter, this is true. However, ratios are general in nature and are just as relevant in other health care settings. For example, use of a current ratio which measures an entity's liquidity is valid and helpful not only for hospitals, but for nursing homes, health maintenance organizations, outpatient clinics, and surgi-centers. Furthermore, understanding the application of financial ratios in the relatively more complex hospital environment makes their application in other settings easier.

LIQUIDITY RATIOS

Liquidity is a term frequently used by business and financial people. It refers to the ability of a firm to meet its short-term maturing obligations. The more liquid a firm, the better it is able to meet its short-term obligations or current liabilities. Liquidity is an important dimension in the assessment of financial condition. Most firms that experience financial problems do so because of a liquidity crisis: they are unable to pay current obligations as they become due. Measuring an entity's liquidity position is *central* to determining its financial condition. Other long-term factors, such as a poor accounts receivable collection policy, may explain a poor liquidity position but the worsening of a liquidity position is usually the first clue that something more basic is wrong.

Current Ratio

One of the most widely used measures of liquidity is the current ratio which equals

$$\frac{\text{Current Assets}}{\text{Current Liabilities}}$$

For Willkram Hospital, the current ratio values for 1976 and 1975 are as follows:

1976	*1975*
$\dfrac{7,326}{2,833} = 2.586$	$\dfrac{6,201}{2,669} = 2.298$

The higher the ratio value the better the firm's ability to meet its current liabilities. A value commonly used in industry as a standard is 2.00; this means that two dollars of current assets (assets expected to be realized in cash during the year) are available for each one dollar of current liabilities (obligations expected to require cash within the year). A standard value derived from a sample of American Hospital Association (AHA) members is 2.5. On both a trend and a standard comparison basis, Willkram Hospital is in a favorable position. (See Exhibit 4-3).

The current ratio is a basic measure and is widely used. However, if used alone it does not tell the whole story. Some types of assets, cash and marketable securities for example, are more liquid than accounts receivable or inventory. The current ratio does not account for these differences.

Quick Ratio

Another liquidity ratio that is a refinement of the current ratio is the quick ratio which equals

$$\frac{\text{Current Assets Less Inventory}}{\text{Current Liabilities.}}$$

For Willkram Hospital, the quick ratio values for 1975 and 1976 are:

1976	*1975*
$\dfrac{7326 - 682}{2833} = 2.345$	$\dfrac{6201 - 578}{2669} = 2.107$

As with the current ratio, the higher the value of this ratio the better the firm's liquidity position. In industry, a value of 1.0 is often used. However this value is too low for health care facilities because such a small amount of their current asset investment is carried in inventory. A value of 2.16 is the 1976 average for the AHA sample and is used here as our standard. On both a trend and a standard comparison basis, Willkram Hospital is in a favorable position.

In the quick ratio, the numerator is largely composed of cash and marketable securities plus accounts receivable. These current assets are more liquid and make this a better test of liquidity than the current ratio. However, a key assumption is the liquidity of the accounts receivable. If they are not being collected quickly because of poor collection policies or delays in third party payment processing, the quick ratio may not be a good measure of liquidity.

Acid Test Ratio

A refinement of the quick ratio is the acid test ratio which equals

$$\frac{\text{Cash Plus Marketable Securities}}{\text{Current Liabilities.}}$$

For Willkram Hospital, the acid test ratios for 1976 and 1975 are as follows:

1976	*1975*
$\frac{119}{2833} = .042$	$\frac{67}{2669} = .025$

Higher values again indicate more liquid resources available to meet current liabilities coming due. In this case the liquid assets are limited to cash and marketable securities. Both these assets could be liquidated with little or no delay to pay maturing current liabilities. In the quick and current ratios there are categories of current assets that cannot be converted into cash without significant delays. A standard value derived from the AHA sample is .18. We shall use this value as our standard. Willkram Hospital has a favorable trend but an unfavorable relationship to this standard value. In short, Willkram Hospital appears to be underinvested in highly liquid assets like cash and marketable securities, but its trend over the two-year period is favorable.

All three of the previous ratios—current, quick and acid test—give indexes of the liquidity position of an entity. They do not, however, provide information as to *why* the current liquidity position exists, or what can be done to change it.

Days in Accounts Receivable

Days in accounts receivable is a liquidity ratio that indicates possible cause for a worsening liquidity position. It is simply ending net accounts receivable divided by an average day's revenue.

$$\frac{\text{Net Accounts Receivable}}{\text{Total Operating Revenue}/365}$$

For Willkram Hospital, days in accounts receivable for 1976 and 1975 were as follows:

1976	*1975*
$\dfrac{\dfrac{5732}{31,311}}{365} = 66.819$	$\dfrac{\dfrac{5147}{26,916}}{365} = 69.797$

Values for this ratio indicate the number of days in the average collection period. For example, Willkram Hospital in 1976 had 66.82 days outstanding in accounts receivable at the year end. This implies that it took the hospital 66.82 days on the average to turn its accounts receivable into cash. High values for this ratio could indicate problems in collection time that may be due to the collection policies and billing systems of the entity. However, a high value might also indicate that the underlying quality of the accounts receivable is poor, i.e., their collectibility may be in doubt. This might imply that the write-off policy of the entity should be reexamined.

A good way to evaluate the collectibility of accounts receivable is to perform an aging of accounts receivable by payor. For example, let's assume that the following aging of Willkram's accounts receivable as of December 31, 1976 was performed.

WILLKRAM HOSPITAL
AGING OF ACCOUNTS RECEIVABLE
December 31, 1976
(In Thousands)

	Gross	Self-Pay	Third Party
Less than 30 Days	$3,000	$ 800	$2,200
31–90 Days	1,800	300	1,500
91–365 Days	500	300	200
Over 365 Days	1,300	700	600
Total	$6,600	$2,100	$4,500

The above aging of accounts receivable casts doubt on the collectibility of many of the $700,000 self-pay accounts receivable over one year past due. It might also raise a question of why $600,000 of third party payor receivables over one year are still outstanding. The answer could be a poor collection policy for payment by third parties such as Medicaid, or an unresolved dispute between the providor and the payor over the amount actually due.

Standard values for this ratio are readily available in the hospital industry. They are not as readily available in other sectors of the health care industry, however. For our purposes we have chosen a standard value of 62 days, a figure published by the American Hospital Association based on an extensive sampling of its member hospitals. Willkram Hospital has a favorable trend in days in accounts receivable but an unfavorable comparison against the standard value. This could be part of the reason that Willkram's acid test ratio is low. For example, if the collection period were sped up by three days, (the difference between Willkram's current collection period and the standard), an additional $257,000 in cash could be collected. If this potential cash balance were added to the present cash value of $119,000, the acid test ratio value would be raised to .133. This represents a 316% improvement over its current value.

Care must be exercised in using any of the liquidity ratios if seasonality is a factor. For example, if the dates for financial statement presentation occur during a slack period of the year, certain values of current assets may be understated and others overstated. In particular the values of accounts receivable and inventory might be at their lowest point of the year, and the corresponding values of cash and marketable securities at their highest or vice versa, giving a biased view of the liquidity position of the firm. In addition, standards vary by type of health care facility and region of the country. Clinics and health maintenance organizations can be expected to have significantly fewer days in accounts receivable than normal hospitals would maintain, while long-term care facilities may have significantly longer collection periods than normal hospitals. The collection period also depends heavily upon the composition of payers and their payment practices. Medicaid may pay on a prompt and timely basis in one state and yet be delinquent in another. The same holds true for Blue Cross and other major third party payers.

Payables Index

Another index that provides some information about causes of a worsening liquidity position is the Payables Index:

$$\frac{\text{Current Liabilities}}{\text{(Total Operating Expenses} - \text{Depreciation)}}$$

For Willkram Hospital the values of this ratio for 1976 and 1975 are as follows:

1976	*1975*
$\dfrac{2833}{\dfrac{(30{,}774 - 1944)}{365}} = 35.9$	$\dfrac{2669}{\dfrac{(26{,}358 - 1880)}{365}} = 39.8$

From a financial condition standpoint, low values of this ratio are better than higher values. Creditors often use a slight adaption of this ratio—

$$\frac{\text{Accounts Payable}}{\dfrac{\text{Purchases}}{365}}$$

If the data is available, both ratios should be calculated. In the Willkram Hospital example no separate lising of purchases for the year is available. The payables index ratio indicates the length of time an entity takes to pay its obligations. The denominator, which is total expenses less depreciation divided by 365, provides an index of average daily cash expenses. (Remember, depreciation is a noncash expense.) The numerator, current liabilities, represents obligations for expenditures during the coming year. Most normal supply items are expensed within the year in which they are purchased. The same is true for payroll expenses, which usually constitute the largest single element of accrued liabilities and expenses. A standard value for this ratio derived from the AHA sample is 37.2. On this basis, Willkram Hospital has both a favorable trend and standard comparison.

Day's Cash on Hand

A final measure of liquidity is day's cash on hand:

$$\frac{(\text{Cash} + \text{Marketable Securities})}{\dfrac{(\text{Total Operating Expenses} - \text{Depreciation})}{365}}$$

For Willkram Hospital, the values of day's cash on hand for 1976 and 1975 are as follows:

1976	*1975*
$\dfrac{119}{\dfrac{(39{,}774 - 1944)}{365}} = 1.51$	$\dfrac{67}{\dfrac{(26{,}358 - 1880)}{365}} = .999$

Higher values of this ratio imply a more liquid position, other factors remaining constant. The ratio measures the number of days an entity could meet its average daily expenditures (as measured by the denominator) with existing liquid assets, namely cash and marketable securities. It is similar to the acid test ratio except that it uses a flow rather than stock concept. It attempts to define a maximum period of safety assuming the worst of all conditions, e.g., no conversion of accounts receivable into cash.

In one study of hospital financial statements,* the average value for this ratio was ten. With ten as a standard, Willkram Hospital is acutely underinvested in cash and marketable securities, although its trend is favorable. The value of this ratio in conjunction with the value of the acid test ratio strongly implies that Willkram Hospital should seriously consider increasing the amount of cash and marketable securities, especially marketable securities, that it carries. This is the only area where liquidity position is in drastic need of improvement.

Capital Structure Ratios

Capital structure ratios are useful in assessing the long-term solvency or liquidity of a firm. While the liquidity ratios just discussed are useful in detection of immediate solvency problems, the capital structure ratios are especially useful in longer-term assessment of financial condition. They are also valuable in detecting some short-term problems. Capital structure ratios are carefully evaluated by long-term creditors and bond rating agencies to determine an entity's ability to increase its amounts of debt financing. In the last twenty years the hospital and health care industries have radically increased their percentages of debt financing. This trend makes capital structure ratios vitally important to many individuals. Evaluation of these ratios may well determine the amount of credit available to the industry and thus directly affect its rate of growth.

Fund Balance to Total Assets

One basic capital structure ratio is the fund balance to total assets ratio:

$$\frac{\text{Fund Balance}}{\text{Total Assets}}$$

---

*R. Thompson, "Ratio Analysis in the Hospital Industry," unpublished master's thesis, Ohio State University, 1976.

For Willkram Hospital the values for this ratio in 1976 and 1975 are as follows:

<table>
<tr><td><u>1976</u></td><td><u>1975</u></td></tr>
<tr><td>$\dfrac{21,026}{43,492}$ = .483</td><td>$\dfrac{20,415}{41,808}$ = .488</td></tr>
</table>

Higher values for this ratio are regarded as positive indicators of a sound financial condition, all other things being equal. After all, if an entity had zero debt or a Fund Balance to Total Assets ratio of one, there would not be any possible claimants on the entity's assets and thus no fear of bankruptcy or insolvency. The ratio indicates the percentage of total assets that has been financed with sources other than debt. In industry a value for this ratio of less than fifty percent can cause some alarm. In segments of the health care industry where there is greater stability in earnings, lower ratios may be permitted. In fact, a rule of thumb used by some investment bankers in the hospital industry is a value of .35 or better. Using this value as our standard, Willkram Hospital has a favorable position on both a trend and a standard comparative basis. This might indicate that more debt could be handled satisfactorily.

Long-Term Debt to Fund Balance

Another capital structure ratio used by many analysts is the long-term debt to fund balance ratio:

$$\frac{\text{Long-Term Debt}}{\text{Fund Balance}}$$

For Willkram Hospital, the values for this ratio in 1976 and 1975 are as follows:

<table>
<tr><td><u>1976</u></td><td><u>1975</u></td></tr>
<tr><td>$\dfrac{19,633}{21,026}$ = .934</td><td>$\dfrac{18,724}{20,415}$ = .917</td></tr>
</table>

One deficiency of the fund balance to total asset ratio is that it includes short-term sources of debt financing, such as current liabilities. When assessing solvency, and the ability to increase long-term financing, it is sometimes desirable to focus on "permanent capital." Permanent capital consists of sources of financing which are not temporary, including long-term debt and fund balance. Low values for the long-term debt to fund balance ratio indicate to creditors an entity's ability to carry additional long-term debt.

A value used in general industry is 50%; that is, for every one dollar of long-term debt, two dollars should come from equity. In the health care industry this value may be higher, especially for hospitals. A value used by many investment bankers is 2.0. In other words they are willing to allow two dollars of long-term debt for every one dollar of equity. In part this reflects the stability of the industry. It also reflects the relative difficulty in acquiring equity capital in a largely nonprofit industry. Based on a standard value of 2.00, Willkram Hospital has a slightly unfavorable trend but a highly favorable standard comparison. Once again, Willkram Hospital appears capable of financing significant future capital expansion with debt financing.

Long-Term Debt to Fixed Assets

A capital structure ratio of special importance to the health care industry is the long-term debt to fixed asset ratio:

$$\frac{\text{Long Term Debt}}{\text{Fixed Assets}}$$

For Willkram Hospital the values for this ratio in 1976 and 1975 are as follows:

1976	*1975*
$\frac{19,633}{34,806} = .564$	$\frac{18,724}{34,414} = .544$

This ratio's use in credit evaluations of cost reimbursed health care entities, especially hospitals, is increasing. The higher the value of this ratio, the worse the financial condition of the entity.

To see the importance of this ratio, imagine a health care entity with 100% of its patients on a cost reimbursement formula—cash flow in this situation would equal depreciation, because revenues would be set equal to expenses. Since repayment of debt principal is not an expense, as we discussed in the last chapter, creditors would look to the cash flow of the entity for repayment. The long-term debt to fixed asset ratio represents the relationship between need for cash flow to repay outstanding debt principal and available cash flow or undepreciated fixed assets.

No standard value is readily available for this ratio. Assuming that long-term debt may be repaid in approximately 50% of the life of the financed assets, a value of .50 can be used as a hypothetical standard. Imagine a four-year life asset with a cost of $1,000 that is financed with $500 of two-year notes and $500 internal funds. The notes will be retired in equal installments in each of the first two years. If cash flow is limited to depreciation, the following pattern of net cash flow will emerge:

Year	1	2	3	4
Depreciation	$250	$250	$250	$250
Less Debt Retirement	250	250	-0-	-0-
Net Cash Flow	-0-	-0-	$250	$250

With this value of .50 as a standard, Willkram Hospital has both an unfavorable trend and an unfavorable standard comparison. Although neither is severe, each might limit debt financing capability in the future because the major source of cash flow, namely fixed assets, may not be adequate in some creditor's minds. At a minimum, Willkram Hospital's condition might imply a need to negotiate for longer debt repayment plans in any future financing programs.

Times Interest Earned

A traditional capital structure ratio that attempts to measure the ability of an entity to meet its interest payment is the times interest earned ratio:

$$\frac{\text{Excess of Revenues over Expenses plus Interest Expense}}{\text{Interest Expense}}$$

For Willkram Hospital, the values for this ratio in 1976 and 1975 are as follows:

1976	*1975*
$\frac{597 + 1403}{1403} = 1.426$	$\frac{752 + 1514}{1514} = 1.497$

Even though a firm has a very low percentage of debt financing, it may not be able to carry additional debt because its profitability cannot meet the increased interest payment. Repayment of interest expense is a very important consideration in long-term financing. Failure to meet interest payment requirements on a timely basis could result in the entire principal value of the loan becoming due. Meeting the fixed annual interest expense obligations is thus highly critical to solvency. The times interest earned ratio measures the extent to which earnings could slip and still not impair the entity's ability to repay its interest obligations. High values of this ratio are obviously preferable. An absolute minimum standard in general industry is 1.5. Compared to this standard, Willkram Hospital shows both an unfavorable trend and an unfavorable standard comparison. Since this ratio indicates the ability to repay indebtedness, Willkram's low value could seriously impair its ability to acquire additional financing on favorable terms.

Debt Service Coverage

A commonly used capital structure ratio that measures the ability to pay both components of long-term indebtedness—interest and principal—is the debt service coverage ratio:

$$\frac{\text{Excess of Revenues over Expenses plus Depreciation plus Interest}}{\text{Principal Payment plus Interest Expense}}$$

In the financial statements of Willkram Hospital available to us, there are no data we can use to calculate values for this ratio since the amount of principal repayments is missing. However, values for debt principal repayments in 1976 and 1975 can be identified in the footnote to the financial statements (which are not reprinted here). Using these values, debt service coverage ratios for Willkram Hospital in 1976 and 1975 are as follows:

1976		*1975*	
$\frac{597 + 1944 + 1403}{850 + 1403}$	$= 1.75$	$\frac{752 + 1880 + 1514}{800 + 1514}$	$= 1.79$

The debt service coverage ratio is a broader measure of debt repayment ability than the times interest earned ratio since it includes the second component of a debt obligation—the repayment of debt principal. The numerator of the debt service coverage ratio defines the funds which are available to meet debt service requirements of principal and interest. The ratio then indicates the number of times that the debt service requirements can be met from existing funds. Higher ratios indicate that an entity is obviously better able to meet its financing commitments.

A standard debt service coverage ratio value used by investment bankers in the hospital industry is 1.5. With this value as a standard, Willkram Hospital has a slightly unfavorable trend and a favorable standard comparison. This may at first seem to contradict the conclusion reached in the analysis of the times interest earned ratio, where an unfavorable standard comparison existed. However, the favorable comparison in the debt service coverage ratio results from a currently favorable depreciation to principal repayment ratio. Specifically, depreciation in 1976 is 2.28 times the debt principal repayment in that year. If future depreciation charges are reduced or debt principal retirement payments increased, there could be some future problems. However, at the present time this ratio is favorable and seems to indicate that Willkram Hospital could obtain additional debt financing if needed.

Activity Ratios

Activity or turnover ratios measure the relationship between revenue and assets. The numerator is always revenue, and may be thought of as a surrogate measure of output; the denominator is investment in some category of assets, and may be thought of as a measure of input. These ratios are also referred to as efficiency ratios, since efficiency ratios measure output to input. As we will discuss later, activity ratios also have a very important relationship to measures of profitability.

Total Asset Turnover

The most widely used turnover ratio is total asset turnover:

$$\frac{\text{Total Operating Revenue}}{\text{Total Assets}}$$

For Willkram Hospital, the values of the total asset turnover ratio in 1976 and 1975 are as follows:

1976	*1975*
$\frac{31,311}{43,492} = .720$	$\frac{26,916}{41,808} = .644$

A high value for this ratio implies that the entity's total investment is being used efficiently, that a large number of services is being provided to the community from a limited resource base. However, the ratio can be deceptive. For example, a facility that is relatively old, with most of its plant assets fully depreciated, is quite likely to show a high total asset turnover ratio. Yet it may not be nearly as efficient as a newer facility that has plant and equipment assets which are largely undepreciated.

A measure that may be partially used to evaluate the existence of this problem by detecting the age of a given physical plant is

$$\frac{\text{Allowance for Depreciation}}{\text{Depreciation}} = \text{Average Age of Facility.}$$

Using this measure for Willkram Hospital, the values for 1976 and 1975 are as follows:

1976	*1975*
$\frac{8368}{1944} = 4.30$	$\frac{6474}{1880} = 3.44$

The calculated values of these ratios imply that Willkram Hospital operates in a relatively new facility. Specifically, at December 31, 1976 the plant of Willkram Hospital appears to be approximately 4.3 years old.

Though the values for the total asset turnover ratio may be deceptive, a standard value of 1.2 has been reported in several studies of hospital financial statements. By this standard, Willkram Hospital has a favorable trend but a highly unfavorable standard comparison. Much of this could be due to the relative newness of the facility.

Fixed Asset Turnover

Another common turnover ratio is the fixed asset turnover ratio:

$$\frac{\text{Total Operating Revenue}}{\text{Fixed Assets}}$$

For Willkram Hospital, the values of the fixed assets turnover ratios in 1976 and 1975 are as follows:

1976	*1975*
$\frac{31,311}{34,806} = .900$	$\frac{26,916}{34,414} = .782$

The fixed asset turnover ratio is identical to the total asset turnover ratio, except that fixed assets, a specific subset of total assets, is substituted in the denominator. This substitution is an attempt to assess the relative efficiency of an individual category of assets. In fact, all the additional turnover ratios that will be discussed later are further segregations of various categories of assets.

Fixed assets are the number one investment in most health care entities. The fixed asset ratio can thus be of major importance in assessing the relative efficiency of plant investments. A standard value of 1.75 has been reported in one study of hospital financial statements* and will be used for our purposes. Once again, Willkram Hospital shows a favorable trend but an unfavorable standard comparison. As this facility becomes older, the value of its fixed asset turnover ratio will probably approach the standard value. In most situations, there are better ways to assess the efficiency of plant investment than by using this very simple ratio, by actual measures of utilization for example. However, an aggregated measure of cost like that used in a fixed asset turnover ratio does provide important information with respect to output per dollar of investment.

Current Asset Turnover

The complement of the fixed asset turnover ratio is the current asset turnover ratio:

$$\frac{\text{Total Operating Revenue}}{\text{Current Assets}}$$

For Willkram Hospital, the values of this ratio in 1976 and 1975 are as follows:

1976	*1975*
$\frac{31,311}{7,326} = 4.274$	$\frac{26,916}{6,201} = 4.341$

This ratio focuses on the relative efficiency of the investment in current assets with respect to the generation of revenue. The valuation of current assets is not subject to the same difficulties encountered in the measurement of fixed assets. The ratio is thus more comparable across facilities. The value of the standard for this ratio is 4.0, based on the AHA sample. Willkram Hospital has a slightly unfavorable trend and a slightly favorable standard comparison.

---

*M. Choate, "Financial Ratio Analysis," *Hospital Progress* (January 1974).

Accounts Receivable Turnover

A refinement of the current asset turnover ratio is the accounts receivable turnover ratio:

$$\frac{\text{Total Operating Revenue}}{\text{Net Accounts Receivable}}$$

For Willkram Hospital the values of this ratio in 1976 and 1975 are as follows:

1976	*1975*
$\frac{31,311}{5,732} = 5.462$	$\frac{26,916}{5,147} = 5.229$

The major purpose of this ratio is to break down investment further. A low current asset turnover ratio might indicate an overinvestment in current assets, but it would not pinpoint in which categories of current assets the overinvestment occurred. There is a similarity between this ratio and the days in accounts receivable ratio discussed in the liquidity section. In fact, the accounts receivable turnover ratio can be derived by dividing 365 by the value of days in accounts receivable. The standard value for this ratio of 5.89 is derived by dividing 365 by 62, the standard value for days in accounts receivable. The conclusions reached from the evaluation of accounts receivable turnover are identical to those reached in days in accounts receivable. Willkram Hospital has a favorable trend, but it does appear to be overinvested in accounts receivable.

Inventory Turnover

Another refinement of the current asset turnover ratio is the inventory turnover ratio:

$$\frac{\text{Total Operating Revenue}}{\text{Inventory}}$$

For Willkram Hospital, the values of this ratio in 1976 and 1975 are as follows:

1976	*1975*
$\frac{31,311}{682} = 45.91$	$\frac{26,916}{578} = 46.57$

The inventory turnover ratio is a very important measure of financial condition in manufacturing and merchandising firms. Low values might imply overstocking of items that are not selling. Conversely, a high value could also indicate that inadequate inventory levels may be reducing possible sales because of shortages. In service firms like health care facilities, inventory is of less importance. However, it still is a major category of current asset investment, and its relative efficiency is important. Using a standard value of 50*, derived from a published study of hospital financial statements, Willkram Hospital exhibits an unfavorable trend and an unfavorable standard comparison. Although neither is serious, the hospital might investigate their current level of inventory.

Profitability Ratios

To talk of profit in a largely nonprofit industry appears to many to be a contradiction in terms. The important point is that few, if any, health care facilities can remain liquid and solvent if profits are held zero. Cash flow would not be sufficient to meet normal nonexpense cash flow requirements, such as repayment of debt principal and investment in additional fixed and current assets.

Recognizing the basic need for profit is not the same thing as determining how much is needed. It is not healthy for the public, or a health care entity, if the entity's profitability is either too great or too small. Discussion of what creates a need for profitability centers on a definition of financial requirements. This will be addressed in the next chapter. Here we are concerned only with the interpretation of several commonly used financial ratios of profitability.

Operating Margin

A frequently used financial ratio of profitability is the operating margin ratio:

$$\frac{\text{Net Operating Income}}{\text{Total Operating Revenue}}$$

---

*M. Choate, "Financial Ratio Analysis," *Hospital Progress* (January 1974).

For Willkram Hospital, the values of this ratio in 1976 and 1975 are as follows:

$$\underline{1976} \qquad\qquad \underline{1975}$$

$$\frac{537}{31,311} = .017 \qquad\qquad \frac{558}{26,916} = .021$$

From the entity's viewpoint, the higher the value of the ratio the better its financial condition. In most situations, firms that have high profit margins are less likely to experience financial difficulties than those which do not. A simple way to understand this ratio is to think of it as a measure of profit retained per dollar of sales. For example, in 1976 Willkram Hospital retained 1.7¢ of every revenue dollar as profit. A standard value published by the American Hospital Association for an extensive sample of hospitals in 1976 is .025. Thus Willkram Hospital shows both an unfavorable trend and an unfavorable standard comparison. This evaluation may indicate that Willkram's rate structure should be reexamined in light of a relatively low operating margin.

There are several deficiencies in the interpretation of this ratio that should be discussed. First, this ratio uses net operating income, not the excess of revenues over expenses, as its measure of profitability. Some health care facilities receive significant sums of money from sources other than operations, such as investment from endowments and contributions. To the extent that they are available, these funds may be used to subsidize operations. If we replace net operating income with excess of revenues over expenses in the numerator, the margin ratios for Willkram Hospital in 1976 and 1975 now become:

$$\underline{1976} \qquad\qquad \underline{1975}$$

$$\frac{597}{31,311} = .019 \qquad\qquad \frac{752}{26,916} = .027$$

Some problems might still exist in Willkram Hospital's profitability, but they are less severe when the values of nonoperating income are indicated.

Second, return per dollar of sales or operating margins is only one view of profitability. The ultimate question is whether the level of profit is sufficient in relationship to the investment. Operating margin ratios do not directly assess this.

Return on Total Assets

A profitability ratio that does measure the relationship of profit to investment is the return on total assets ratio:

$$\frac{\text{Net Operating Income}}{\text{Total Assets}}$$

For Willkram Hospital, the values of this ratio in 1976 and 1975 are as follows:

1976	*1975*
$\dfrac{537}{43,492} = .012$	$\dfrac{558}{41,808} = .013$

There is an important relationship between (1) the return on total asset ratio, (2) the product of the operating margin ratio, and (3) the total asset turnover ratio:

(1)		(2)		(3)
$\dfrac{\text{Net Operating Income}}{\text{Total Assets}}$	$=$	$\dfrac{\text{Net Operating Income}}{\text{Total Operating Revenue}}$	$\times$	$\dfrac{\text{Total Operating Revenue}}{\text{Total Assets}}$

Return on total assets is thus the product of the operating margin ratio and the total asset turnover ratio. Improvement in the operating margins of individual services through increased prices or reduced costs will improve the return on total assets of the entity as a whole. Also, a reduction in investment or an increase in revenue, while investment is held constant, will also improve the return on total assets ratio by increasing the total assets turnover ratio.

The standard value which we will use for the return on total asset ratio is .03. This is derived by simply multiplying our standard value for the operating margin ratio—.025—times the standard total asset turnover ratio value of 1.2. Naturally, Willkram Hospital again has an unfavorable standard comparison and a slightly unfavorable trend. Both the operating margin ratio and the total asset turnover ratio values are below the standards. While the total asset turnover ratio will probably improve as the facility becomes older and more of its cost is depreciated, the same is not necessarily true for the operating margin ratio. It thus appears that a priority for Willkram Hospital should be a thorough investigation of both rates and costs of individual service and product lines.

Again, it is possible to use the excess of revenues over expenses as the numerator in the return on total asset ratio. The values for 1976 and 1975 are as follows:

1976	1975
$\dfrac{597}{43,492} = .014$	$\dfrac{752}{41,808} = .018$

Nonoperating Revenue to Excess of Revenues over Expenses

A profitability ratio that provides a means of analyzing the source of profit is the nonoperating revenue to excess of revenue over expenses ratio:

$$\frac{\text{Nonoperating Revenue}}{\text{Excess of Revenues over Expenses}}$$

For Willkram Hospital, the values for this ratio in 1976 and 1975 are as follows:

1976	1975
$\dfrac{60}{597} = .101$	$\dfrac{194}{752} = .258$

Depending on the individual situation, a high value for this ratio may be good or bad. A high value would indicate that a large percentage of total net income or excess of revenues over expenses was derived from sources other than operations. If the value is stable, it enhances the overall financial condition of the entity and provides a stable source of funding that could be used to meet temporary reversals in operations. However, a high value may also indicate a weak financial condition. For example, there are many health care facilities that are heavily dependent on nonoperating revenue sources to subsidize operations that by themselves are incapable of breaking even. If these sources are not guaranteed, and exhibit a highly erratic pattern, the financial condition of the entity could be in jeopardy. Selecting a standard value for this ratio is not easy or necessarily meaningful. In the case of Willkram Hospital, there is a significant change in the proportion of income contributed by nonoperating revenue sources from 1975 to 1976. During this same period, net operating income was fairly stable. A longer-term trend analysis could reveal the importance of this change in nonoperating revenue. Given Willkram Hospital's low profitability ratio values, the sources of nonoperating revenue and their expected stability should be analyzed.

Excess of Revenue over Expenses to Changes in Fund Balance

Given the peculiar nature of fund accounting in the hospital and health care industry, another valuable profitability ratio is the Excess of Revenue over Expenses to Changes in Fund Balance ratio.

$$\frac{\text{Excess of Revenue over Expenses}}{\text{Change in Fund Balance}}$$

For Willkram Hospital, the values for this ratio in 1976 and 1975 are as follows:

1976		*1975*	
$\dfrac{597}{(21,026 - 20,415)}$	$= .977$	$\dfrac{752}{(20,415 - 19,242)}$	$= .641$

As we discussed in Chapter 3, there are situations where funds may be transferred to an unrestricted fund from a restricted fund and not be shown as income to the unrestricted fund. An important example of this occurrence is the purchase of fixed assets with dollars from a restricted plant replacement fund. The fixed assets purchased would be transferred to the unrestricted fund and shown as general plant property and equipment; a corresponding direct charge or increase in fund balance of the unrestricted fund would also occur. This increase in fund balance is necessary if the basic accounting equation is to be kept in balance: assets must equal liabilities plus fund balance. If this situation occurs frequently, the financial condition of the entity is far more favorable than its profitability ratios would indicate. Therefore, the ratio of excess of revenue over expenses to changes in fund balance is designed to determine to what extent such transactions are occurring. Values consistently, and significantly, less than one indicate that a very important, unreported source of income is being used by the entity.

Once again, selecting a standard value for this ratio is not necessarily meaningful or relevant. In a case of Willkram Hospital, a significant source of unreported income occurred in fiscal year 1975: reported income or the excess of revenues over expenses accounted for only 64.1% of the total change in fund balance. A history of such situations could imply a much more favorable financial condition than current profitability ratios might indicate. For example, if the change in fund balance were used as a measure of income in the operating margin ratio, the value of that ratio for 1975 would become .044. This is significantly higher than the standard of .025 and indicates a dramatically changed financial condition.

SUMMARY

In this chapter we discussed the use of financial ratio analysis in the assessment of the financial condition of health care facilities. Calculation of the 20 ratios defined in this chapter aid this process immeasurably. There are, however, some general limitations that should be recognized when evaluating financial condition through financial ratio analysis.

Validity of Standards

The standards used in this chapter should be helpful in many health care settings. They are, however, of special importance in the hospital industry since that is where they were derived. These ratios will vary by region of the country and time period. This implies that standards should be updated frequently. It also implies the importance of using adequate trend data. Financial ratios should be calculated over a minimum of five years if meaningful trends are to be discovered. The two-year comparisons developed in this chapter are not adequate and were used only to discuss basic methodology.

Cost Valuation

The values reported in a balance sheet are usually stated at unadjusted historical cost. While this valuation does have some advantages in terms of objectivity of reporting, it limits the utility of comparisons across facilities when inflation is a predominant factor. The need for adjustment of ratios that use balance sheet values, especially fixed asset values, *cannot be overstated.*

Projections

Financial ratio analysis uses historical data. It provides a picture of where the entity has been; it does not necessarily tell where it is going. Budgetary data is required for this purpose. The value of financial ratio analysis as a predictor rests on the assumption that past behavior validly indicates future behavior.

Accounting Alternatives

It should be recognized that a number of acceptable accounting alternatives exist for measuring the financial effects of various transactions. Use of different accounting methods can create significantly different values for financial ratios, even when the underlying financial events are identical; consistent use of given accounting methods erases many comparability problems that might be created. However, there may be situations where differences in accounting methods may impair the comparability of financial ratios among individual health care facilities and over time.

Exhibit 4-1

Willkram Hospital Balance Sheet Unrestricted Funds, December 30, 1976 (with comparative figures for 1975) (In Thousands)

ASSETS		December 31, 1976	December 31, 1975
Current Assets			
Cash & marketable securities		$ 119	$ 67
Accounts receivable	$6,600		$5,900
Less allowances & uncollectibles	868		753
Net accounts receivable		5,732	5,147
Inventories		682	578
Prepaid expenses		397	177
Due from restricted fund		396	232
TOTAL CURRENT ASSETS		$ 7,326	$ 6,201
Property, plant & equipment			
Construction in progress		104	125
Property, plant & equipment		43,070	40,763
		43,174	40,888
Allowances for depreciation		8,368	6,474
Total Property, Plant & Equipment		34,806	34,414
Other (Board Restricted) Investments		1,360	1,193
TOTAL ASSETS		$43,492	$41,808

Exhibit 4-1 continued

LIABILITIES AND FUND BALANCE	December 31, 1976	December 31, 1975
Current Liabilities		
Accounts Payable	$ 1,472	$ 1,265
Notes Payable	0	250
Due to Third Party	310	188
Accrued Expenses	708	611
Due to Restricted Funds	343	355
Total Current Liabilities	2,833	2,669
Long-term debt		
Mortgage payable	19,633	18,724
Total Liabilities	22,466	21,393
Fund Balance	21,026	20,415
TOTAL LIABILITIES AND FUND BALANCE	$43,492	$41,808

Exhibit 4-2

Willkram Hospital Statement of Revenues and Expenses, Year Ended December 31, 1976 (with comparative figures for 1975) (In Thousands)

	1976	1975
Patient Services Revenue	$31,824	$27,177
Allowances and Uncollectible Accounts	1,934	1,411
Net Patient Service Revenue	29,890	25,766
Other Operating Revenue	1,421	1,150
TOTAL OPERATING REVENUE	31,311	26,916
Operating Expenses		
Nursing Services	9,306	7,364
Medical Services	7,907	6,523
General Services	5,285	5,271
Administrative Services	3,683	2,780

Exhibit 4-2 continued	1976	1975
Education and Research	1,246	1,026
Depreciation	1,944	1,880
Interest	1,403	1,514
TOTAL OPERATING EXPENSES	30,774	26,358
Net Operating Income	537	558
Nonoperating Revenue	60	194
EXCESS OF REVENUES OVER EXPENSES	$ 597	$ 752

Exhibit 4-3

Financial Ratio Analysis of Willkram Hospital

				EVALUATION	
RATIO	1976	1975	STANDARD	TREND	STANDARD
Liquidity					
1. Current	2.586	2.298	2.50	Favorable	Favorable
2. Quick	2.345	2.107	2.16	Favorable	Favorable
3. Acid Test	.042	.025	.18	Favorable	Unfavorable
4. Days in Accounts Receivable	66.82	69.80	62.00	Favorable	Unfavorable
5. Days Cash on Hand	1.510	.999	10.00	Favorable	Unfavorable
6. Payables Index			37.20	Favorable	Favorable
Capital Structure					
1. Fund Balance to Total Assets	.483	.488	.35	Favorable	Favorable
2. Long-Term Debt to Fund Balance	.934	.917	2.00	Unfavorable	Favorable
3. Long-Term Debt to Fixed Assets	.564	.544	.50	Unfavorable	Unfavorable
4. Times Interest Earned	1.426	1.497	1.5	Unfavorable	Unfavorable
5. Debt Service Coverage	1.75	1.79	1.5	Unfavorable	Favorable
Activity					
1. Total Asset Turnover	.720	.644	1.20	Favorable	Unfavorable
2. Fixed Asset Turnover	.900	.782	1.75	Favorable	Unfavorable
3. Current Asset Turnover	4.274	4.341	4.00	Unfavorable	Favorable

Exhibit 4-3 continued

4. Accounts Receivable Turnover	5.462	5.229	5.89	Favorable	Unfavorable
5. Inventory Turnover	45.91	46.57	50.00	Unfavorable	Unfavorable

Profitability

1. Operating Margin	.017	.021	.025	Unfavorable	Unfavorable
2. Return on Total Assets	.012	.013	.03	Unfavorable	Unfavorable
3. Nonoperating Revenue to Excess of Revenue over Expenses	.101	.258	NA	NA	NA
4. Excess of Revenue over Expenses to Change in Fund Balance	.977	.641	NA	NA	NA

NA = Not Available.

Chapter 5

Cost Concepts and Decision Making

In the last three chapters we have focused on understanding and interpreting the financial information prepared by the financial accounting system and presented in general purpose financial statements. This chapter is directed more narrowly at the utilization of cost information in decision making. Cost information is produced by the cost accounting system of an entity. In most situations, it is shaped by the financial accounting system and the generally accepted principles of financial accounting. However, it is more flexible, since it usually provides information for identifiable and specific decision-making groups such as budgetary cost variance reports to department managers, cost reimbursement reports to third party payers, and forecasted project costs to health systems agencies.

Cost is a noun that never really stands alone. In most situations, two additional pieces of information are added which enhance the meaning and relevance of the cost statistic.

First, the object being costed is defined. For example, we might say that the cost of routine nursing care in Willkram Hospital was $100. Objects of costing are usually of two types:

1. products (outputs or services)
2. responsibility centers (departments or larger units)

Quite often we oversimplify this classification system and refer to cost information about products as *planning information* and cost information about responsibility centers as *control information.*

Secondly, usually an adjective is added to modify cost. For example, we might say that the direct cost of routine nursing care in Willkram Hospital was $100. A number of major categories of adjective modifiers refine the concept of cost; they are all used to improve the decision-making process by precisely defining cost to make it more relevant to decisions.

This chapter will discuss some of the basic concepts of cost used in cost analysis. It is important to explain this jargon if decision makers are to use cost information correctly. Different concepts of cost are required for different decision purposes. In most situations, these concepts require specific, unique methodologies for cost measurement.

CONCEPTS OF COST

Cost may be categorized in a variety of ways to meet decision makers' specific needs. However, in most situations the total value of cost is the same. Using one cost concept in place of another simply slices the total cost pie differently. For example, in Exhibit 5-1, the total cost of the laboratory for June 1977 was $21,360. Of that amount, $20,000 could be classified as direct cost and $1,360 as indirect cost. However, classifying costs by controllability might determine that $15,000 of the laboratory cost was controllable and $6,360 was not controllable. The total cost, however, is the same in both cases.

This brings us to another important point. Since in most cases different concepts of cost simply slice total cost in different ways, there may be underlying relationships between the various concepts of costs. For example, direct costs and controllable costs may be related. In many situations there are standard rules of thumb that may be used to relate cost measures.

The difference between cost and expense is another crucial definitional point. Accountants have traditionally defined cost in a way that leads one to think of cost as an expenditure. However, in most reported cost statistics, the definition is usually one of expense and not necessarily expenditure. For example, in Exhibit 5-1, depreciation is listed as a cost. However, depreciation is not an actual expenditure of cash but an amortization of prior cost. Unless otherwise indicated, when we are discussing cost statistics the term costs and expenses may be used interchangeably.

For purposes of discussion, we will examine four major categories within which costs can be classified:

- traceability to the object being costed
- behavior of cost to output or activity
- management responsibility for control
- time period for which costs are computed

Traceability

Of all cost classifications, traceability is the most basic. Two major categories of costs classified by traceability are (1) direct costs and (2) indirect costs. A direct cost is specifically traceable to a given cost objective. For example, the salaries, supplies and other costs of Exhibit 5-1 are classified as direct costs of the laboratory. Indirect costs cannot be traced to a given cost objective without resorting to some arbitrary method of assignment. In Exhibit 5-1, depreciation, employee benefits and costs of other departments would be classified as indirect costs.

Not all costs classified as indirect may actually be indirect. There are some situations where they could be redefined as direct costs. For example, it might be possible to calculate employee benefits for specific employees; these costs could then be charged to the departments where the employees worked and thus become direct costs. However, the actual costs of performing these calculations might be prohibitive.

The classification of a cost as either direct or indirect depends on the given cost objective. This is a simple observation, but one that is forgotten by many users of cost information. For example, the $20,000 of direct cost identified in Exhibit 5-1 is a direct cost, only with respect to the laboratory department. If another cost objective is specified, the cost may no longer be direct. For example, dividing the $20,000 of direct costs by the number of relative value units yields a direct cost per relative value unit of $2.00. But, this is not really true. The direct cost of any given relative value unit may be higher or lower than the $2.00 calculated, which is the average value for all relative value units and not necessarily the cost for any specific unit.

Incorrect classification is a common problem in cost accounting. Costs are accumulated on a department or responsibility center basis, and may be direct or indirect with respect to that department. However, it can be misleading to say that the same set of direct costs is also direct with respect to the outputs of that department.

Direct cost categories of most departments would include the following three major categories:

- salaries
- supplies
- other (usually fees and purchased services such as utilities, dues, travel and rents)

Indirect cost categories usually include—

- depreciation
- employee benefits
- allocated costs of other departments

The concept of direct versus indirect cost may not appear to have much specific relevance to decision makers. To some extent this is true, however, the concept of direct versus indirect costs is *pervasive*. It influences both the definition and measurement of other alternative cost concepts which do have specific relevance.

Cost Behavior

Cost is also classified by the degree of variability in relation to output. The actual measurement of cost behavior is influenced by department's classifications of cost, which provides the basis for categorizing costs as direct or indirect.

For our purposes, we will identify four major categories of costs that are classified according to their relationship to output:

1. variable
2. fixed
3. semifixed
4. semivariable

Variable costs change as output or volume changes in a constant, proportional manner. That is, if output increases by 10%, costs should also increase by 10%—there is some constant cost increment per unit of output. Exhibit 5-2 illustrates, graphically and mathematically, the concept of variable cost for the laboratory example of Exhibit 5-1. It is assumed that all supply costs in this case are variable. For each unit increase in relative value units, supply costs will increase by 50¢.

Fixed costs do not change in response to changes in volume. They are a function of the passage of time, not output. Exhibit 5-3 illustrates fixed cost behavior patterns for the depreciation costs of the laboratory example. Each month, irrespective of output levels, depreciation cost will be $160.

Semifixed, or step, costs do change with respect to changes in output, but they are not proportional. A semifixed cost might be considered variable or fixed—depending on the size of the steps relative to the range of volume under consideration. For example, in Exhibit 5-4, it is assumed that the salaries cost of the laboratory are semifixed. If the volume of output under consideration for a specific decision were between 6,000 and 8,000 relative value units, salary costs could be considered fixed at $9,000. Some semifixed costs may be considered variable for cost analysis purposes. For example, if smaller units of people could be employed instead of full-time equivalents, such as hours generated by an available part-time pool, the size of the steps might be significantly smaller in our laboratory example than 2,000 relative value units. At the present it is assumed that one additional FTE must be employed for every increment of 2,000 relative work units. Treating salary costs as variable in this situation might not be a bad assumption.

Semivariable costs include an element of both fixed and variable costs; utility costs are good examples. There may be some basic, fixed requirement per unit of time, (month, year, etc.) regardless of volume, such as normal heating and lighting requirements. But there is also likely to be a direct, proportional relationship between volume and the amount of the utility cost. As volume increases, costs do go up. Exhibit 5-5 illustrates semivariable costs in the case of the laboratory.

In many situations, we do not focus on specific cost elements, but aggregate several cost categories of interest. It is interesting to see what type of cost behavior pattern emerges when we do. Exhibit 5-6 aggregates the four cost categories discussed earlier—supplies, depreciation, salaries and other. A semi-variable cost behavior pattern very closely approximates the actual aggregated cost behavior pattern; this is true for many types of operations. In the next section we will discuss some very simple but useful methods for approximating this cost function.

Controllability

One of the primary purposes of cost information is to aid the management control process. To facilitate evaluation of the management control process, costs must be assigned to individual responsibility centers, usually departments, where a designated manager is responsible for cost control. A natural question that arises is what proportion of the total costs charged to a department is the manager responsible for? The answer to this question implies a need to categorize costs into two categories: controllable costs and noncontrollable costs.

Controllable costs can be influenced by a designated responsibility or departmental manager within a defined control period. It is often said that all costs are controllable by someone at some time. For example, the chief executive officer of a health care facility, through the authority granted to him by his governing board, is ultimately responsible for all costs.

The following matrix of costs uses the laboratory's cost report of Exhibit 5-1. All of the allocated costs are assumed to be broken down as follows:

LABORATORY COST EXAMPLE
Cost Behavior

Trace-ability	Variable	Fixed	Semi-Fixed	Total
Direct	Other $4,000 Supplies 5,000 $9,000	Other $1,000	Salaries $10,000	$20,000
Indirect	Employee Benefits $150 House- keeping $100 _____ $250	Deprecia- tion $160 Adminis- tration $500 House- keeping $100 $760	Mainte- nance $250 Laundry $100 $350	$1,360
	TOTAL $9,250	$1,760	$10,350	$21,360

All costs must fall into one of the above six cells, however, it may be possible to categorize an aggregated cost category into more than one cell. In the laboratory example, other cost was viewed as semivariable, implying that part of the cost would be described as a direct variable cost ($4,000) and part as a direct fixed cost ($1,000).

There is a tendency in developing management control programs, especially in the health care industry, to use one of three approaches in designating controllable costs. First, controllable costs may be defined to be the total costs charged to the department: the department manager would view all costs in the above six categories as controllable. All $21,360 of cost would be viewed as controllable by the laboratory manager. In most normal situations, this grossly overstates the amount of cost actually controllable by a given departmental manager. The result of this overstatement has been negative in many situations. Departmental managers have rightfully viewed this basis of control as highly inequitable.

Second, another concept of controllable costs would limit controllable cost to those costs classified as direct. This system is also not without fault: specifically, there may be fixed costs attributed directly to the department that should not be considered controllable. Rents on pieces of equipment for example, may not be under the departmental manager's control. There may also be indirect costs, especially costs which are variable, that department manager can control. For example, employee benefits may legitimately be under the department manager's responsibility.

Third, in some situations, controllable costs are defined as only those costs which are direct/variable. This limits costs which are controllable by the department manager to their lowest level. However, it excludes what could be a relatively large amount of cost influenced by the department manager. Failure to include these costs in the manager's control sphere may weaken management control.

Future Costs

Decision making involves selection among alternatives; it is a forward looking process. Actual historical cost may be useful to project future costs, but it should not be used without adjustment unless it can be assumed that future conditions will be identical to the past.

A variety of cost concepts and definitions have been used in current discussion of costs for decision making purposes. We will discuss four that are basic to selecting among alternative decisions.

1. avoidable costs
2. sunk costs
3. incremental costs
4. opportunity costs

Avoidable costs will be affected by the decision under consideration. Specifically, they are costs that can be eliminated or saved if an activity is discontinued, and will continue only if the activity is left unchanged. For example, if a hospital were considering curtailing its volume by 50% in response to cost containment pressures, what would it save? The answer is those costs which are avoidable. In most situations, multiplying current, average, total cost per unit of output (patient days or admissions) by the projected change in output would overstate avoidable costs; a considerable proportion of the cost may be classified as sunk.

Sunk costs are unaffected by the decision under consideration. In the example above, large portions of cost, depreciation, administrative salaries, insurance and others, are sunk or not avoidable to the proposed 50% reduction in volume.

The distinction between fixed and variable costs and sunk and avoidable costs is not perfect. Many costs which are classified as fixed may also be thought of as sunk, but some are not. For example, malpractice insurance premiums may be generally considered fixed cost given an expected normal level of activity. However, if the institution is considering a drastic reduction in volume, malpractice premiums may not be entirely fixed.

Incremental costs are the changes in total cost resulting from various alternatives of action. Avoidable costs may be thought of as a subset of incremental costs, but most people use the term avoidable costs to refer to the comparison of cost where one alternative is reduction in volume or discontinuation of some activity. Incremental costs usually refer to situations where the alternative is an expansion of volume or the initiation of a new activity. For decisions involving only modest changes in output, incremental costs and variable costs may be used interchangeably. In most situations, incremental costs are more comprehensive. A decision to construct a surgi-center adjacent to a hospital would involve fixed and variable costs. Depreciation on the facility would be a fixed cost but it would be incremental to the decision to construct the surgi-center.

Opportunity cost is the value foregone by using a resource in a particular way instead of in its next best alternative usage. Assume that a nursing home is considering expanding its facility and would use land acquired twenty years ago. If the land had a historical cost of $1,000,000, but a present market value of $10,000,000, what is the opportunity cost of the land? Practically everyone would agree that if sale of the land constituted the next best alternative, the opportunity cost would be $10,000,000, not $1,000,000. Alternatively, a hospital might consider converting part of its acute care facility into a skilled nursing facility because of a reduction in demand or obsolescence in the facility. The question arises, what is the value or what would the cost of the facility be to the skilled nursing facility operation? If there is no way that the facility can be renovated or if the facility is not needed for the provision of acute care, its opportunity cost may be zero. This could contrast sharply to the recorded historical cost of the facility.

COST MEASUREMENT

This section will discuss methods of cost measurement for two cost categories: direct and indirect or full cost, and variable and fixed cost.

Both of these costs concepts are useful in financial decisions, but the cost accounting system does not directly provide estimates for them.

Full Cost

In most cost accounting systems, costs are classified by department or responsibility center or by object of expenditure. Costs are classified primarily along departmental lines. Individual cost items are charged to the departments to which they are traceable. Costs are also classified by object of expenditure, whether the expense was for supplies, salaries, rent, insurance or other.

Departments in a health care facility can be classified generally as direct or indirect departments, based on whether they provide services directly to the patient or not. Sometimes the terms revenue and nonrevenue are substituted for direct and indirect. In the hospital industry, the following breakdown is used in general purpose financial statements.

Operating Expense Area	Type of Department
Nursing Services Area	direct/revenue
Other Professional Services	direct/revenue
General Services	indirect/nonrevenue
Fiscal Services	indirect/nonrevenue
Administrative Services	indirect/nonrevenue

Whatever the nomenclature used to describe the classification of departments, cost allocation is a fundamental need. The costs of the indirect, nonrevenue departments need to be allocated to the direct revenue departments for many decision making purposes. For example, third party payers usually reimburse on the basis of the full costs of direct departments and are interested only in the cost of indirect departments as far as they affect the calculation of the direct departments' full costs. Pricing decisions also need to be based on full costs, not just direct costs, if the costs of the indirect departments are to be covered equitably.

Equity is a key concept in allocating indirect department costs to direct departments. Ideally, the allocation should reflect as nearly as possible the actual cost incurred by indirect departments to provide services for a direct department. Department managers who receive cost reports showing indirect allocations are vitally interested in this equity argument, and for good reason. Even if indirect costs are not regarded as controllable by the department manager, the allocation of costs to a given direct department can have an important effect on a variety of management decisions. Pricing is an important one, expansion or contraction of department, purchase of new equipment and salaries of departmental managers are also affected by the allocation of indirect costs.

Costs of indirect departments are in most cases not traceable to direct departments. If they were, they could be reassigned. They must be allocated to direct departments in some systematic and rational manner. In general, two allocation decisions must be made: selection of the allocation basis, and selection of the method of cost apportionment.

Exhibit 5-7 provides data for a sample cost allocation. There are four departments: Two indirect—laundry and linen, and housekeeping; and two are direct—radiology and nursing. Pounds of laundry is the only allocation basis under consideration for the laundry and linen department. The housekeeping department can use one of two allocation bases, either square feet of area served or hours of service actually worked.

In general, there are only three acceptable methods of cost allocation:

1. step down
2. double distribution
3. simultaneous equations

Most health care facilities still use the step down method of cost allocation. In this method, the indirect department that receives the least amount of service from other indirect departments and provides the most service to other departments allocates its cost first. A similar analysis follows to determine the order of cost allocation for each of the remaining indirect departments. This determination can be subjective and allows some flexibility which we shall see shortly.

In the step down allocation process illustrated below, laundry and linen allocates its cost first. Then, housekeeping allocated its direct cost, plus the allocated cost of laundry and linen, to the direct departments of radiology and nursing on the ratio of services provided to those departments. The allocation proportions are given in parentheses.

	Direct Costs	Laundry	Housekeeping	Total
Laundry	$15,000	$15,000		
Housekeeping	30,000	750(.05)	$30,750	
Radiology	135,000	750(.05)	9,711(.3158)	$145,461
Nursing	270,000	13,500(.90)	21,039(.6842)	304,539
Total	$450,000	$15,000	$30,750	$450,000

The order of departmental allocation can be an important variable in a step down method of cost allocation. Shown below is the alternative cost allocation when housekeeping allocates its cost first and preceeds laundry and linen.

	Direct Costs	Housekeeping	Laundry	Total
Housekeeping	$30,000	$30,000		
Laundry	15,000	1,500(.05)	$16,500	
Radiology	135,000	9,000(.30)	868(.0526)	$144,868
Nursing	270,000	19,500(.65)	15,632(.9474)	305,132
Total	$450,000	$30,000	$16,500	$450,000

The double distribution method of cost allocation is just a refinement of the step down method. Instead of closing the individual department after allocating its costs, it is kept open and receives the costs of other indirect departments. After one complete allocation sequence, these departments are then closed by using the normal step down method. The simultaneous equation method of cost allocation is an attempt to be exact about the cost allocation amounts. A system of equations is established and mathematically correct allocations are computed. In the above example, if simultaneous equations had been used, the cost of radiology would be $145,075 and the cost of nursing would be $304,925.

Finally, using a different allocation base can create differences in cost allocation. For example, using the square footage basis for housekeeping, instead of hours served, produces the following pattern of cost allocation when housekeeping allocates its cost first in the step down method:

	Direct Cost	Housekeeping	Laundry & Linen	Total
Housekeeping	$30,000	$30,000		
Laundry & Linen	15,000	7,500(.25)	$22,500	
Radiology	135,000	1,500(.05)	1,184(.0526)	$137,684
Nursing	270,000	21,000(.70)	21,316(.9474)	312,316
TOTAL	$450,000	$15,000	$22,500	$450,000

The important point in this discussion is that full cost is not as objective and exact a figure as one might normally think. Indirect costs can be allocated in a variety of ways which can create significant differences in full costs for given departments. This flexibility should be remembered when examining and interpreting full cost data.

Variable and Fixed Costs

A very important and pervasive cost concept is variability with respect to output. It is involved in determining costs such as avoidable, sunk, incremental, and controllable for decision making. However, accounting records do not directly yield this type of cost information. Instead, costs are classified by department and by object of expenditure. In order to develop estimates of variable and fixed costs, this data must be analyzed in some way.

The discussion of cost concepts classified by variability with respect to output disclosed that a semivariable cost pattern may be a good representation of many types of costs. A semivariable cost function is one that has both a fixed and variable element in it, especially when various types of costs are aggregated together, such as total department costs, total facility costs or even aggregations of minor cost elements like salaries and wages at the department level.

Estimation of a semivariable cost function requires separation of cost into variable and fixed components. A variety of methods, varying in complexity and accuracy, may be used. Three of the simplest methods are (1) visual fit, (2) high-low, and (3) semi-averages.

To illustrate each of these three methods, assume that we are trying to determine the labor cost function for the radiology department and we have the following six biweekly payroll data points:

Pay Period	Number of Films	Hours Worked
1	300	180 (low)
2	240	140 (low)
3	400	230 (high)
4	340	190 (high)
5	180	110 (lowest)
6	600	320 (highest)

In the visual fit method of cost estimation, the individual data points are plotted on graph paper. A straight line is then drawn through these points to provide the best fit. Visual fitting of data is a good first step in any method of cost estimation. Below is a visual fitting of the radiology data:

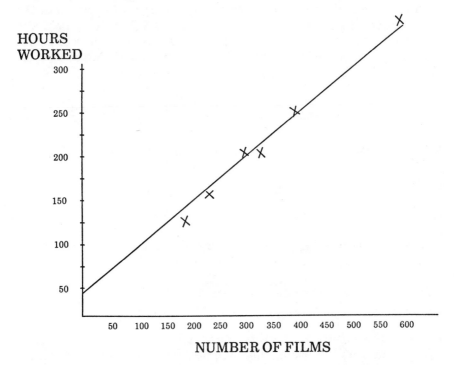

The high-low method is a simple method that can be used to estimate the variable and fixed cost coefficients of a semivariable cost function. The variable cost parameter is solved first and equals the change in cost from the high to the low data point, divided by the change in output. In the radiology example

$$\text{Variable Labor Hours/Film} = \frac{320-110}{600-180} = \frac{210}{420} = .50$$

The fixed cost parameter may then be solved by subtracting the estimated variable cost (determined by multiplying the variable cost parameter estimate times output at the high level) from total cost. In the case of the radiology example, fixed cost would equal

Fixed Labor Hours/biweekly pay period = $320 - (.50 \times 600) =$
$$320 - 300 = 20$$

Alternatively, it is also possible to plot the high and low points and then draw a straight line through them.

The semiaverages method is very similar to the high-low method, in terms of its mathematical solution. The difference in cost from the mean of the high cost points and the mean of the low cost points is divided by the change in output from the mean of the high cost points and the mean of the low cost points to derive the estimate of variable cost. In the radiology example, variable cost would be

$$\text{Variable Labor Hours/Film} = \frac{320+230+190}{3} - \frac{180+140+110}{3} =$$

$$\frac{\dfrac{600+400+340}{3} - \dfrac{300+240+180}{3}}{}$$

$$\frac{246.67 - 143.33}{446.67 - 240.00} = .50$$

Fixed cost is solved in a manner identical to the high-low method. In the radiology example, fixed cost would equal

Fixed Labor Hours/biweekly pay period = $246.67 - (.50 \times 446.67) =$
$$23.34$$

These three methods of estimating variable and fixed cost are highly simplistic. They are useful only in limited ways to provide a basis for further discussing and analyzing what the true cost behavioral pattern might be. However, in most situations a limited attempt, based on simplistic methods, to discover the underlying fixed/variable cost patterns, is better than no effort.

When these methods are used, several data checks should be performed. First, the cost data being used to estimate the cost behavior pattern should be stated in a common dollar. If the wages paid for employees have changed dramatically from one year to the next, using unadjusted wage and salary data from two years can create measurement problems. In the radiology example, we used a physical quantity measure of cost, namely hours worked. A physical measure of cost should be used whenever it can. Second, cost and output data should be matched; the figures for reported cost should relate with the activity of the period. In most situations, accounting records do provide this type of relationship because of the accrual principle of accounting. However, in some situations this may not be true: supply costs may be charged to a department when the items are purchased, and not necessarily when they are used. Third, the period of time during which a cost function is being estimated should be one of a stable technology and case mix. If the technology under consideration has changed dramatically during that period, there will be measurement problems.

COST-VOLUME-PROFIT ANALYSIS

There are certain techniques that can be applied in analyzing the relationship between cost, volume and profit. These techniques rely on categorizing cost into fixed and variable. The techniques themselves are powerful management decision aids that may be valuable in a wide range of decisions. Understanding of these techniques is also valuable for decision makers whose choices affect the financial results of health care facilities.

For example, profit in a health care facility is influenced by factors that include—

- rates
- volume
- variable cost
- fixed cost
- reimbursement formulas
- bad debts

The primary value of cost-volume-profit analysis, or breakeven analysis as it is sometimes called, is its ability to quantify the relationships between these factors and profit.

Traditional Breakeven Analysis

Breakeven analysis has been used in industry for decades with a high degree of satisfaction. Its name comes from the solution to an equation that sets profit equal to 0, with revenue set equal to costs. To illustrate breakeven analysis we will use the following example. Assume that a hospital has the following relevant financial information:

Variable Cost Per Day	$40.00
Fixed Cost Per Period	$6,000.00
Rate Per Day	$120.00

The breakeven volume may be solved by dividing fixed costs by the contribution margin, which is the difference between rates and variable cost.

$$\text{Breakeven in Units} = \frac{\text{Fixed Cost}}{\text{Contribution Margin Per Unit}}$$

In our sample hospital, breakeven would be

$$\text{Breakeven in Units} = \frac{\$6,000}{\$120 - \$40} = 75 \text{ Patient Days.}$$

If volume exceeds 75 patient days, the hospital will make a profit, but if it goes below 75 units it will incur a loss. Sometimes, individuals graph a revenue and cost relationship to illustrate profit at various levels. This presentation is referred to as the breakeven chart and is presented in Exhibit 5-8.

In many cases, some targeted level of net income or profit is desired. The breakeven model just presented is easily adapted and the new breakeven point would become

$$\text{Breakeven in Units} = \frac{\text{Fixed Cost} + \text{Targeted Net Income}}{\text{Contribution Margin}}$$

For our sample hospital, assuming that a desired profit of $800 were required, the new breakeven point would be

$$\text{Breakeven in Units} = \frac{\$6,000 + \$800}{\$120 - \$40} = 85 \text{ Patient Days.}$$

Cost Reimbursement and Breakeven Analysis

One of the deficiencies with using traditional breakeven analysis in the health care industry is that it does not reflect the presence of cost reimbursement. The revenue function of hospitals, nursing homes and many other health care facilities is not as simple as that of our previous example. Only a small percentage of patients may actually pay charges, while the majority have their cost reimbursed by a third party payer. A breakeven point may be easily determined. The new breakeven point in a situation of cost reimbursement is

$$\text{Breakeven in Units} = \frac{\text{Fixed Cost} + \dfrac{\text{Desired Net Income}}{\text{Proportion of Charge Paying Patients}}}{\text{Contribution Margin}}$$

If our sample hospital has 80% of its patients on cost reimbursement formulas, its new breakeven point becomes

$$\text{Breakeven in Patient Days} = \frac{\$6,000 \ + \dfrac{\$800}{.2}}{\$120 - \$40} = 125 \text{ Patient Days}$$

This is a substantial increase in volume from the previous level of 85 without incorporating the effect cost reimbursement. It illustrates simply the impact of an increasing level of cost reimbursement on a health care facility. All other things remaining constant, a health care facility faced with an increasing percentage of cost reimbursement must attempt to increase its volume, especially in noncost-reimbursed areas. We will discuss the impact of cost reimbursement in more detail shortly.

This brings us naturally to the pricing question. In most situations, a health care facility reacts to an expected level of volume and tries to provide the necessary services for that patient demand. One of the benefits of breakeven analysis is the derivation of a pricing rule. For the sample cost-reimbursed entity, the recoverable price (the price received from charge paying patients after deducting allowances) must be set equal to the entity's average cost plus its desired level of profit, divided by the number of charge patients:

$$\text{Recoverable Price} = \frac{\text{Variable Cost} + \text{Fixed Cost}}{\text{Expected Volume}} + \frac{\text{Desired Net Income}}{\text{Expected Volume} \times \text{Proportion of Charge Patients}}$$

In the case of our hospital example, if we assume that expected volume is 75 patients and that 80% of these will be covered by cost reimbursement formulas, the recoverable rate must be set equal to

$$\text{Recoverable Price} \ = \ \frac{\$40 \times 75 + \$6,000}{75} + \frac{\$800}{75 \text{x.}2} \ =$$

$$\$120 + \$53.33 = \$173.33$$

One more adjustment must be made before the pricing analysis is complete. Our recoverable rate reflects the average amount recovered from charge patients; in fact, rates must be established at a higher level to reflect the probability of doubtful accounts and other allowances. To adjust this rate to reflect the rate that must actually be charged, the recoverable rate must be divided by one minus the proportion of charge patient revenue that is ultimately written off:

$$\text{Established Rate} \ = \ \frac{\text{Recoverable Rate}}{1 - \begin{array}{c} \text{Proportion of} \\ \text{Charge Revenue} \\ \text{Written Off} \end{array}}$$

For the sample hospital, if we assume that 20% of all charge revenue is written off, the established rate would be

$$\text{Established Rate} \ = \ \frac{173.33}{1 - .2} \ = \ \$216.67$$

If this hospital charged $216.67 per patient day, the hospital would just meet its desired profit level of $800. This can be seen from the statement of revenues and expenses which follows:

Patient Services Revenue (75 × $216.67)	$16,250
Less Contractual Allowances (216.67 − $120.00) × 60)	5,800
Doubtful Accounts (15 × .2 × $216.67)	650
Net Patient Services Revenue	9,800
Less Fixed Costs	6,000
Variable Costs (75 × $40)	3,000
Excess of Revenues Over Expenses	$ 800

The impact of cost reimbursement on pricing is important. To some extent, it has gone unnoticed by many individuals charged with the responsibility of examining hospital and health care prices, including individuals both inside and outside the industry. The preceding analysis shows that what you charge is not necessarily what you collect. For example, the study hospital would charge $216.67 per patient day, but would collect $120 per patient day from its cost payers (probably including Medicare, Medicaid, and Blue Cross). The following graph illustrates the relationship between rates and the percentage of cost reimbursement:

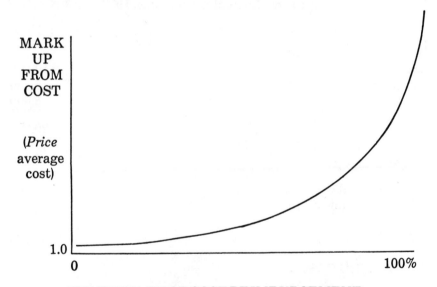

PERCENTAGE OF COST REIMBURSEMENT

For those patients unfortunate enough not to have a third party payer, the reality of the above graph does not need to be pointed out. A national health insurance plan that reimbursed health care providers on the basis of cost could certainly accelerate charges dramatically. Individuals who have no insurance and commercial insurance carriers who generally pay charges would be hit with astronomical increases in rates. In short, as the percentage of cost-reimbursed patients increases, the gap between rates and costs escalates.

SUMMARY

Cost accounting systems provide different measures of cost for different decision making purposes. This is a desirable objective and is not to be viewed as an exercise in number playing. To understand what measure of cost is needed for a specific decision, a user must have some knowledge about cost and the variety of alternative concepts of costs. The terms covered in this chapter should be useful in helping decision makers define their needs more precisely.

Exhibit 5-1

Cost Report Laboratory, for June, 1977

DIRECT COSTS

Salaries	$10,000
Supplies	5,000
Other	5,000
TOTAL	$20,000

DEPRECIATION

Building and Fixed Equipment	100
Major Movable Equipment	60
TOTAL	160

ALLOCATED COSTS

Employee Benefits	150
Administration	500
Maintenance	250
Housekeeping	200
Laundry	100
TOTAL	1,200

TOTAL COSTS	$21,360
RELATIVE VALUE UNITS (RVU) PRODUCED	10,000
AVERAGE COST PER RVU	$ 2,136

Exhibit 5-2

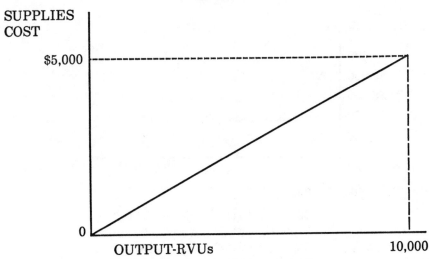

Cost Behavior of Supplies Cost
Variable

SUPPLIES
COST

$5,000

0

OUTPUT-RVUs   10,000

Supplies Cost = $.50 × Number of RVUs

Exhibit 5-3

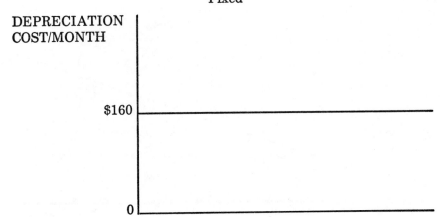

Cost Behavior of Depreciation
Fixed

DEPRECIATION
COST/MONTH

$160

0

OUTPUT-RVUs

Depreciation Cost = $160 per month

Exhibit 5-4

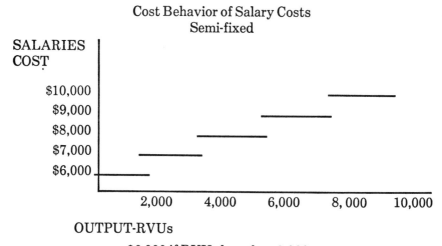

Cost Behavior of Salary Costs
Semi-fixed

$6,000 if RVUs less than 2,000
$7,000 if RVUs between 2,001 and 4,000
Salary Costs = $8,000 if RVUs between 4,001 and 6,000
$9,000 if RVUs between 6,001 and 8,000
$10,000 if RVUs between 8,001 and 10,000

Exhibit 5-5

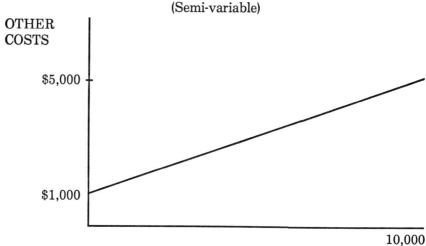

Cost Behavior of Other Costs
(Semi-variable)

Other Costs = $1,000 per month + $.40 × RVUs

Exhibit 5-6

Cost Behavior Aggregated Costs (Direct Cost and Depreciation)

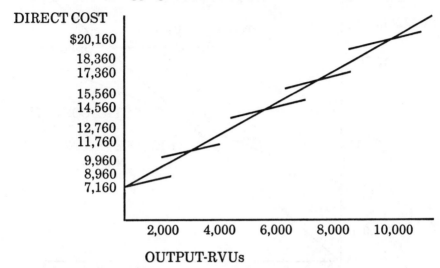

OUTPUT-RVUs

Direct Cost and Depreciation = $7,160 per month + $1.30 × RVUs
(approximation)

Exhibit 5-7

Cost Allocation Example

Department	Direct Costs	Pounds of Laundry Used	Square Feet	Hours of Housekeeping Used
Laundry & Linen	$ 15,000	——	50,000	150
Housekeeping	30,000	5,000	——	——
Radiology	135,000	5,000	10,000	900
Nursing	270,000	90,000	140,000	1,950
	$450,000	$100,000	$200,000	$3,000

Exhibit 5-8

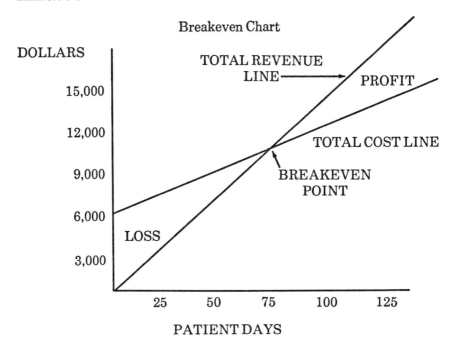

Breakeven Chart

Chapter 6

The Management Control Process

The word budgeting was not in the vocabulary of many hospital managers and other health care facility administrators twenty years ago. Today, this is no longer true and most hospitals and other health care facilities do develop and use budgets in their overall management control process.

To a large extent, the development of institutional budgets in the health care industry may not have been completely voluntary. Section 234 of Public Law 92-603 requires hospitals, extended care facilities and home health agencies to develop an overall plan and budget that—

1. provides for an annual operating budget that would include budgeted income and expenses;
2. provides for a capital expenditure plan for at least a three-year period that would identify the need for capital expenditures and also the projected sources of financing;
3. provides for a review and updating on an annual basis;
4. is prepared under the general direction of the governing body of the facility by a committee that will consist of representatives of the governing body, the administrative staff and the medical staff, of the facility.

Rate setting agencies also frequently require hospitals and other health care facilities to submit fairly detailed institutional budgets. Health systems agencies also require a projection of financial information for projects that they must review.

External forces certainly stimulated the development of budgets in the health care industry, but most likely budgets would have developed anyway. Hospitals and health care facilities have grown larger and more complex, in organization and finances. Budgeting is a *must* in organizations where management authority is delegated to many individuals.

For our purposes, a budget will be defined as a quantitative expression of a plan of action. It is an integral part of the overall management control process of an organization.

Anthony and Herzlinger* discuss management control in great detail. They define it as follows: "Management control is a process by which managers assure that resources are obtained and used effectively and efficiently in the accomplishment of an organization's objectives."

Efficiency and Effectiveness

In the above definition, great emphasis is placed on attaining efficiency and effectiveness. In short, they determine the success or failure of management control.

These two terms have very precise meanings. Often individuals talk about the relative efficiency and effectiveness of their operations as if the two were identical, or highly correlated. They are not identical, nor are they necessarily correlated. An operation may be effective without being efficient, and vice versa. A well managed operation should *ideally* be both effective and efficient. Efficiency is easier to measure and its meaning is fairly well understood: efficiency is simply a relationship between outputs and inputs. For example, a cost per patient day of $110 is a measure of efficiency; it tells how many resources, or inputs, were used to provide one day of care, the measure of output.

Managers and other persons wishing to assess management in the health care industry are increasing their use of efficiency measures. In most situations, efficiency is measured by comparison to some standard. Several basic preconditions should be identified if efficiency measures are to be used intelligently. First, output measures may generally not be comparable. For example, comparing the costs per patient day of care in a 50-bed rural hospital and in a 1,000-bed teaching hospital is not likely to be meaningful. A day of care in a teaching hospital typically entails more service. Second, cost measures may not be comparable or useful for the specific decision under consideration. For example, two operations may be identical, but one is in a newer facility and would have a higher depreciation charge, or the two account for costs differently. For example, one hospital may use an accelerated depreciation method such as the sum of the year's digits,

---

*Management Control in Nonprofit Organizations (Homewood, Ill.: Richard D. Irwin, 1976).

while the other may use straight line depreciation. Third, the cost concept used may not be relevant to the decision under consideration. For
example, a health systems agency deciding which of two hospitals it
will permit to build a 50-bed expansion should obviously consider cost.
However, comparing the full costs of a day of care in each institution
and selecting the lower one could produce bad results: for this specific
decision, the full cost concept is wrong. Incremental or variable cost is
the relevant cost concept for this decision. The focus of interest is on
what the future additional cost would be, not what the historical
average cost was.

Effectiveness is concerned with the relationship between the
organization's outputs and its objectives or goals. A health care facility's typical goals might include solvency, high quality of care, low cost
of patient care, institutional harmony and growth. Measuring effectiveness is more difficult than measuring efficiency for at least two
reasons. First, defining the relationship between outputs and some
goals is difficult, because many facilities' goals or objectives are not
likely to be quantified. For example, exactly how does an alcoholism
program contribute to quality of care? Still, objectives and goals *can*
usually be stated more precisely in quantitative terms. In fact, they
should be quantified to the greatest extent possible. In the alcoholism
program example, quality scales such as frequency of repeat visits or
new patients treated might be developed. Second, the output must
usually be related to more than one organization goal or objective. For
example, solvency and reasonable cost may be two legitimate objectives for a hospital. Continuing an Emergency Room operation might
affect solvency negatively but positively affect patient treatment
costs. How should decision makers weight these two criteria to determine an overall measure of effectiveness?

Control Unit

Most health care facilities are divided into responsibility centers
where management control is exercised. Organizations generally refer
to these responsibility centers as departments. Exhibit 6-1 presents an
organizational chart of a hospital and its departments.

Usually these departments perform special functions that contribute to overall organization goals, directly or indirectly. They
receive resources or inputs and produce services or outputs.

RESOURCES ⟶ | RESPONSIBILITY CENTER | ⟶ OUTPUTS

Responsibility centers are the focus of management control efforts. Emphasis is placed on the effectiveness and efficiency of their operations. Measurement problems occur when the responsibility structure is not identical to the program structure. Decision makers are frequently interested in a program's total cost. Yet in the case of a burn care program, for example, it is unlikely that all the resources used in the program will be assigned to it directly; the costs of medical support services such as physical therapy, laboratory and radiology, as well as other general and administrative services, will not likely be contained in the burn care unit. Program lines typically run across responsibility center or departmental lines. This necessitates cost allocations for decisions that require program cost information. It should be remembered that where cost allocations are involved, the accuracy of the information as well as its comparability may be suspect. For example, one may be interested in the costs of a burn care program, but those costs must be allocated from various departments or responsibility centers, such as laboratory, radiology and housekeeping.

Responsibility centers vary greatly depending upon the controlling organization. For a regulatory agency, the responsibility center might be an entire health care facility; for a health care facility manager, an individual department; and for a departmental manager, a unit within the department. The only requirement is that a designated person be in charge of the identified responsibility center.

Phases of Management Control

Exhibit 6-2 illustrates the relationship of various phases of the management control process to each other and to the planning process. Management control relies on the existence of goals and objectives in an established organization. Without them, the structure and evaluation of the management control process is incomplete. Poor or no planning usually limits the value of management control. Effectiveness becomes impossible to assess without stated goals and objectives; emphasis can only be placed on measuring and attaining efficiency. Thus, an organization can only assess whether it has produced outputs efficiently; it cannot evaluate the desirability of those outputs.

For the purposes of discussion, we shall identify four phases of management control that Anthony and Herzlinger identify in their book:
1. Programming
2. Budgeting
3. Accounting
4. Analysis and reporting

Programming

Programming is the phase of management control that determines the nature and size of programs an organization will use to accomplish its stated goals and objectives. It is the first phase of the management control process and interrelates with planning. In some cases, the line dividing the two activities may be hard to draw. Programming is usually of intermediate length, three to five years. It lasts longer than budgeting, but shorter than planning.

Programming decisions deal with new and existing programs. The methodology differs for programming in these two areas. For example, programming decisions for new programs involve capital investment or capital budget decision making. We will discuss this process more extensively in Chapter 7. Programming decisions for existing programs are often referred to as zero based review, or zero base budgeting. This topic will be discussed later in this chapter.

For an example of the programming process, assume that a stated objective of a hospital organization is to develop and implement a program of ambulatory care in the community. The programming phase of management control would take this stated objective and evaluate alternative programs to accomplish it, such as a surgi-center, an outpatient clinic, or a mobile health screening unit. After this analysis, a decision to construct a ten room surgi-center on a lot adjacent to the hospital would be a program decision.

Budgeting

Budgeting is the management control phase of primary interest in this chapter. It was defined earlier as a quantitative expression of a plan of action. Budgets are usually stated in monetary terms and cover a period of one year.

The budgetary phase of management control follows the determination of programs in the programming phase. In many cases, no real review of existing programs is undertaken, so the budgeting phase often builds on a prior year's budget, or actual results for existing programs. Proponents of zero base budgeting have identified this as a major shortcoming.

The budgeting phase primarily translates program decisions into terms that are meaningful for responsibility centers. The decision to construct a ten room surgi-center will affect the revenues and costs of other responsibility center such as Laboratory, Radiology, Anesthesiology and Business Office. The effects of program decisions must be carefully and accurately reflected in the budgets of individual responsibility centers.

Budgeting may also change programs. More careful and accurate estimation of revenues and costs may reevaluate prior programming decisions as financially unfeasible. For example, the proposed ten-room surgi-center may be shown, through budget analysis, to produce a significant operating loss. If the hospital cannot or will not subsidize this loss from other sources, programming must be changed. The size of the surgi-center may be reduced from ten rooms to five to make the operation break even.

Accounting

Accounting is the third phase of the management control process. Once programs have been decided on and budgets developed for these programs along responsibility center lines, operations begin. Accounting accumulates and records information on both outputs and inputs during the operating phase.

It is important to note that cost information is provided along both program and responsibility center lines. Responsibility center cost information is used in the reporting and analysis phase to determine compliance with budget projections. Programmatic cost information is used to assess the desirability of continuing a given program at its present size and scope in the programming phase of management control.

Analysis and Reporting

The last phase of management control is analysis and reporting. In this phase, differences between actual costs and budgeted costs are analyzed to determine the probable cause of the deviation and reported to the individuals who can correct it. Successful analysis and reporting rely heavily on the information provided from the accounting phase to break down the deviation into categories which suggest possible cause.

In general, there are three primary causes for differences between budgeted and actual costs:

1. Prices paid for inputs were different than budgeted prices.
2. Output level was higher or lower than budgeted.
3. Actual quantities of inputs used were different from budgeted levels.

Within each of these areas, the problem may come from budgeting or operations. A budgetary problem is usually not controllable; no operating action can be taken to correct the situation. For example, the surgi-center may have budgeted for ten RNs at $1,250 each per month. However, if there were no way to employ ten RNs at an average wage less than $1,300 per month, the budget should be adjusted to reflect this change in expectations. Alternatively, the problem may come from operations and be controllable. Perhaps the nurses of the surgi-center are more experienced and better trained than expected. If this is true, and the mix of RNs originally budgeted is still regarded as appropriate, some action should be taken to change the actual mix over time.

THE BUDGETING PROCESS

Budgeting is an integral part of management control, as we have just seen, which is complex in itself. Many regard it as the primary tool which health care facility managers can use to control cost in their organizations. The objectives of budgetary programs as defined by the American Hospital Association are—

1. to provide a written expression, in quantitative terms, of the policies and plans of the hospital;
2. to provide a basis for the evaluation of financial performance in accordance with the plans;
3. to provide a useful tool for the control of costs;
4. to create cost awareness throughout the organization.

The budgetary process is made of a number of interrelated, separate budgets. Exhibit 6-3 provides a schematic representation of the budgetary process and the relationships that exist between specific types of budgets.

The individuals involved in the budgetary process and their roles vary. In general the following individuals or parties may be involved:

1. governing board
2. chief executive officer
3. controller
4. responsibility center managers
5. budgetary committee

The governing board's involvement in the budgetary process is usually indirect. It provides the goals, objectives and approved programs that are used as the basis for budgetary development. In many cases it formally approves the finalized budget, especially the cash budget and budgeted financial statements. These budgets are critical in assessing financial condition, which is a primary responsibility of the governing board.

The chief executive officer or administrator of a health care facility has overall responsibility for budgetary development. The budget is the administrator's tool in the overall program of management by exception which enables him to direct his attention to only those areas where problems exist.

Controllers often serve as budget directors. Their primary function is facilitation: they are responsible for providing relevant data on costs and outputs, and for providing budgetary forms that may be used in budget development. They are not responsible for either making or enforcing the budget.

Responsibility centers are the focal points for control. Managers of departments should be actively involved in developing budgets for their assigned areas of responsibility, and are responsible for meeting the budgets developed for their areas.

Many large health care facilities use a special budgetary committee to aid in budget development and approval. Typically, this committee is comprised of several departmental managers, headed by the controller or administrator. Using a committee structure like this can help legitimize budgetary decisions that might appear arbitrary and capricious if made unilaterally by management.

The Statistics Budget

Developing the statistics budget is the first step in budgeting. It provides the basis for developing revenue and expense budgets later. Together, these three budgets are sometimes referred to as the operating budget. The objective of the statistics budget is to provide measures of work load or activity in each department or responsibility center for the coming budget period. There are three aspects to this task which will be specifically discussed:

- controllable nature of output
- responsibility for estimation
- problems in estimation methodology

Sales forecasts in many businesses reflect management's output expectations—how much of their product can be sold, given certain promotional efforts. There is some question whether health care facilities can affect their volume of service, at least within the usual budgetary period. In the long run, however, through the development or discontinuation of certain programs, volume may be changed.

Most health care facilities implicitly assume in the development of their statistics budget that they cannot affect their overall volume during the coming budgetary period. Instead they assume that they will provide services to meet their actual demand. This leads to a reliance on past period service levels for forecasting demand. Assuming that demand patterns in the budget period will be similar to prior periods can be a costly mistake. First, forseeable but uncontrollable forces may dramatically alter service patterns. For example, retirement of key medical staff with no replacement could drastically reduce admissions. Second, health care facilities may in fact control service levels in the short run and do so in a way to reduce costs. For example, a hospital may decide to use a preadmission testing program which may reduce average length of stay in the hospital, thus reducing total volume and total cost.

The second issue in the statistics budget is assigning responsibility for developing projected output or workload indicators. Should departmental managers provide this information or should top management provide it to them? In some situations, departmental managers may tend to overstate demand. Overstatement of demand implies a greater need for resources within their own area, and creates potential budgetary slack if anticipated volumes are not realized. Top management's incentive is almost converse: understatement of demand may result in a lower total cost budget and eventually lower total, actual costs. Negotiation often becomes necessary in determining demand for budgetary purposes.

The last area of statistics budget development concerns problems of estimation. In most health care facilities, activity in departments depends on a limited number of key variables such as patient days and outpatient visits.

These two key indicators, measured for prior periods and applied through statistical analysis, can be used to project future departmental activity. The major problem becomes one of accurately forecasting values for these key indicators.

Incorporating seasonal, weekly and daily variations in volume is an important estimation problem. Too often yearly volume is assumed to be equal in each monthly period throughout the year, when it is known this is not true. Recognition of seasonal, weekly and daily patterns of variation can create significant opportunities for cost reduction, especially in labor staffing. Finally, output at the departmental level is often multiple in nature. A department produces more than one type of output; for example, a laboratory may provide literally thousands of different tests. In these situations, a weighted unit of service is needed, such as the relative value units often used in areas like Laboratory and Radiology. It is important to recognize the necessity of developing weighted unit measures in the statistics budget, especially where the mix of services is expected to change. Assume that a hospital is rapidly increasing its volume in outpatient clinics. This expansion in volume will increase activity in many other departments, including Pharmacy. If filling an outpatient prescription requires significantly less effort than an inpatient prescription, use of an unweighted activity measure for prescriptions could provide misleading information for budgetary control purposes. Far more labor than is actually needed might be budgeted.

Expense Budget

With estimates of activity for individual departments developed in the statistics budget, department managers can proceed to develop expense budgets for their areas of responsibility. Expense budgeting is the area of budgeting "where the rubber meets the road." Management cost control efforts are finally reflected in hard numbers which departments must live with, in most cases for the budget period. Major categories of expense budgets at the departmental level include payroll, supplies and other. (These three categories were discussed earlier in Chapter 5.) In some situations, a budget for allocated costs from indirect departments may also be included, although this is usually not done by departmental managers.

In our discussion of expense budgeting, we shall focus on the following four issues of budgeting that are of general interest:

1. length of the budget period
2. flexible or forecast budgets
3. standards for price and quantity
4. allocation of indirect costs

Length of the Budget Period

Generally speaking, there are two alternative budget periods that may be used—*fixed* and *rolling*. Of the two, a fixed budget period is far more frequently used in the health care industry. A fixed budget covers some defined time from a given budget date, usually one year. This contrasts with a rolling budget, where the budget is periodically extended on a frequent basis, usually a month or a quarter. For example, in a rolling budget period with a monthly update, the entity would always have a budget of at least eleven months in front of them. The same is not true in a fixed budget, where at fiscal year end there may only be one week or one month left.

A rolling budget has a number of advantages, but it does require more time and effort and therefore more cost. Among its major advantages are—

1. more realistic forecasts which should improve management planning and control;
2. equalization of workload of budget development over the entire year;
3. improved familiarity and understanding of budgets by departmental managers.

Flexible or Forecast Budgets

Use of a flexible budget versus a forecast budget has received much discussion among health care financial people. At the present time, very few hospitals and other health care facilities use a formal system of flexible budgeting. However, flexible budgeting is a more sophisticated method of budgeting than typical forecast budgeting and is being adopted by more and more health care facilities as they become experienced in the budgetary process.

A flexible budget is a budget that adjusts targeted levels of costs for changes in volume. For example, the budget for a nursing unit operating at 95% occupancy would be different than the budget for that same unit operating at an 80% occupancy. A forecast budget would make no formal differentiation in the allowed budget between these two levels.

The difference between a forecast and a flexible budget is illustrated by the historical data and projected use levels for the laboratory presented in Exhibit 6-4. The forecast levels of volume in relative value units for 1978 is identical to the actual volumes of 1977 except that a 10% growth factor is assumed. The departmental manager using this statistics budget must develop a budget for hours worked for 1978. A very common approach to this task is to assume that past work experience indicates future requirements. In this case, the average hours work required per relative value unit in 1977 was .5061. A common method for developing a forecast budget would be to multiply this value of .5061 times the estimated total workload for the budget period, which is expected to be 72,160, and spread the total product equally over each of the twelve months. This is depicted as the forecast budget in Exhibit 6-5.

A major difference between a flexible and a forecast budget is that a flexible budget must recognize and incorporate underlying cost behavioral patterns. In this specific laboratory example, hours worked might be written as a function of relative value units.

Hours worked = (1400 hours per month) + (.25 × relative value units)

Applying this formula to the budgeted relative value units of 1978 yields the flexible budget presented in Exhibit 6-5.

Two points should be made before concluding our discussion of flexible versus forecast budgeting. First, a flexible budget may be represented as a forecast budget for planning purposes. For example, in the laboratory problem of Exhibit 6-5, the flexible budget would provide an estimated hours worked requirement of 34,837 hours for 1978. However, in an actual control period evaluation, the flexible budget formula would be used. To illustrate this point, assume that the actual relative value units provided in January 1978 were 6,500 instead of the forecasted 6,270. Budgeted hours in the flexible budget would not be 2,967, but 3,025.

$$3025 = 1400 + (25 \times 6500)$$

This value would be compared with the actual hours worked, not the initially forecasted 2,967.

Second, dramatic differences in approved .costs can result under these two methods. Recognizing the underlying cost behavioral patterns can change the estimated resource requirements approved in the budgetary process. In our laboratory example of Exhibit 6-5, the forecast budget calls for 36,516 hours versus the flexible budget hours requirement of 34,837. The difference results from the method used to estimate hours worked. In a forecast budget method, the prior average hours per relative value unit relationship is used. In most situations, average hours or average cost should be greater than variable hours or variable cost. In departments with expanding volume, the estimated requirements for resources could be overstated. The converse may be true in departments with declining volume. In many cases, use of forecast budgeting methods is based on the incorporation of prior average cost relationships. Flexible budgeting methods do not make this error since their use depends on explicit incorporation of cost behavioral patterns which distinctly recognize variable and fixed costs.

Standards for Price and Quantity.

Three factors were identified earlier that can create differences between budgeted and actual costs. They are volume, prices and usage or efficiency. Flexible budgeting is an attempt to improve the recognition of deviations caused by changes in volume. Using standards for prices and wage rates, coupled with standards for physical quantities of usage, is an attempt to improve the recognition of deviations from budget that result from the other two factors.

For example, assume that the flexible budget hours requirement for the laboratory example is still

$$\text{Hours worked} = 1400 + (.25 \times \text{relative value units})$$

Furthermore, assume that the budget wage rate is $9 per hour and the actual relative value units for January 1978 were 6,500. Total payroll cost for hours worked (excluding vacations and sick pay) will be assumed to be $31,000. If the actual hours worked were 3,100, the variance analysis report presented in Exhibit 6-6 would be applicable for the Laboratory Department.

The total unfavorable variance of $3,775 results from a $3,100 unfavorable price variance and a $675 unfavorable efficiency variance. Splitting the variance in this manner helps management quickly identify potential causes. For example, the $3,100 price variance may be due to a negotiated wage increase of $1 per hour. If this is the case, the departmental manager is clearly not responsible for the variance. If, however, the difference is due to an excessive use of overtime personnel, or a more costly mix of labor, then the manager may be held responsible for the difference and should attempt to prevent the problem from occuring again. The unfavorable efficiency variance of $675 reflects excessive use of the labor input during the month in the amount of 75 hours. Explanation for this difference should be made and steps taken to prevent its recurrence.

Standard costing techniques have been used in industry for many years as an integral part of management control. While it is true that input and output relationships may not be as objective in the health care industry as they are in general industry, this does not imply that standard costing cannot be used. In fact, there are many areas of activity within a health care facility that do have fairly specific and precise input-output relationships, such as housekeeping, laundry and linen, laboratory, radiology and many others. Standard costing can prove very valuable for cost control in the health care industry, if properly applied.

Allocation of Indirect Cost

Probably more internal strife has occured in organizations over this one issue than almost any other single budgetary issue. A comment often heard is "Why was I charged $3,000 for housekeeping services last month, when my department didn't use anywhere near the level of service?"

A strong case can be made for not allocating indirect costs in budget variance reports. In most normal situations, the receiving department has little or no control over the costs of the servicing department. Allocation may thus raise questions that should not be raised. While it is true that these indirect costs need to be allocated for some decision-making purposes such as pricing, they are generally not needed for evaluating individual responsibility center management.

However, an equally strong argument can also be made for including these direct costs in the budgets of benefiting departments. They are legitimate costs of the total operation and departmental managers should be aware of them. If departmental managers can influence costs in these indirect areas by their decisions, they should be held accountable for them. For example, maintenance, housekeeping and other indirect costs can be influenced by the decisions of benefiting departments. Ideally, a charge for these indirect services should be established and levied against using departments based on their use. Labeling the cost of indirect areas as totally uncontrollable can stimulate excessive and unnecessary use of indirect services and thus have a negative impact on the total cost control program in an organization.

Revenue Budgets

The revenue budget can be set effectively only after the expense budget and the statistics budget have been developed. The not-for-profit nature of the health care industry demands that revenue be related to budgeted expenses. In addition, much of the total revenue actually realized by a health care facility is directly determined by expenses because of the presence of cost reimbursement formulas.

In this discussion of the revenue budget, we will focus on only one aspect of revenue budget development—pricing or rate setting.

Specifically, we will illustrate the rate setting model discussed in Chapter 5 (pp. 133-134) through an additional example.

Exhibit 6-7 illustrates the rate setting model discussed earlier. Sources of information to define the variables of the model are identified, however, three parameters have no identified source:

- desired profit
- proportion of charge patients
- proportion of charge patient revenue not collected

In many situations departmental indicators for these three values are not available. Instead, institution-wide values or averages are substituted. In many cases this may not be a bad approximation, but some serious inequities can result in departments where the relative proportions of inpatient and outpatient use differ greatly. Typically, departments with high outpatient use experience higher levels of charge reimbursement and higher levels of write-offs on that charge reimbursement, due to the reduced presence of insurance coverage for outpatient types of services. Furthermore, the charge patient reimbursement in inpatient areas may be commercial insurance, subject to smaller write-offs. The following figure illustrates this:

	Department #1	Department #2	Total
Desired Profit	$ 500	$ 500	$ 1,000
Budgeted Expense	$10,000	$10,000	$20,000
Estimated Volume	100	100	—
Percentage Bad Debt	4%	20%	12%
Percentage Charge Patients	20%	60%	40%
Percentage Bad Debt on Charge Patients	20%	33%	30%

In most situations, separate figures for both the percentage of write-offs on charge patients and the percentage of charge reimbursement on a departmental basis are not available. Sometimes the best information available may be the percentage of bad debt write-offs on total revenue for the institution as a whole. In the above example, a 4% write-off on 20% of the patients who pay charges in department #1 implies that 20% of the charge patient revenue in that department is written off. The corresponding figure for department #2 is 33%. Using the above data, and substituting the total or aggregate values for percentage write-offs on charge patients and percentage of charge patients, the following rates would be established:

$$\text{Department \#1 Price} = \frac{\dfrac{\$10,000}{100} + \dfrac{\$500}{100 \times .4}}{1 - .30} = \$160.71$$

$$\text{Department \# 2 Price} = \frac{\dfrac{\$10,000}{100} + \dfrac{\$500}{100 \times .4}}{1 - .30} = \$160.71$$

However, proper reflection of the departmental values would yield the following rates:

$$\text{Department\# 1 Price} = \frac{\dfrac{\$10,000}{100} + \dfrac{\$500}{100 \times .2}}{1 - .2} = \$156.25$$

$$\text{Department\# 2 Price} = \frac{\dfrac{\$10,000}{100} + \dfrac{\$500}{100 \times .6}}{1 - .33} = \$161.69$$

In this case, using aggregate or average values produces an inequitable pricing structure. The price for department #1 was initially overstated while the price for department #2 was initially understated. If equity in rate setting is an objective, reliance on average values can prevent the development of an equitable rate structure along departmental lines. In many cases, these errors may be significant.

Determining a desired level of profit is not easy. In many cases it is a subjective process, made to appear objective through the application of a quantitative profit requirement. For example, desired profit may be arbitrarily set at some percentage of budgeted expenses, such as 2% above expenses or a certain percentage of total investment. However, desired levels of profit can in general be stated as the difference between financial requirements and expenses:

$$\text{Desired Profit} = \text{Budgeted Financial Requirements} - \text{Budgeted Expenses}$$

Budgeted financial requirements are cash requirements that an entity must meet during the budget period. There are four elements that usually comprise total financial requirements:

1. budgeted expenses, excluding depreciation
2. requirements for debt principal payment
3. requirements for increases in working capital
4. requirements for capital expenditures

Budgeted expenses at the departmental level should include both direct and indirect (or allocated) expenses. Depreciation charges are excluded because depreciation is a noncash requirement expense.

Debt principal payments include only the principal portion of debt service due. In some cases, additional reserve requirements may be established which may require additional funding. Interest expense is already included in budgeted expenses and should not be included under this category.

Working capital requirements have been discussed earlier. Maintaining necessary levels of inventory, accounts receivable and precautionary cash balances requires an investment. Changes in the total level of this investment must be funded, either from cash, additional indebtedness or a combination of the two. Planned financing of increases in working capital is a legitimate financial requirement.

Capital expenditure requirements may be of two types. First, actual capital expenditures may be made for approved projects. Those projects not financed with indebtedness require a cash investment. Second, prudent fiscal management requires that funds be set aside and invested to meet the reasonable requirements for future capital expenditures. This amount should be related to the replacement cost depreciation of existing fixed assets.

A logical question is how is the desired profit requirement allocated to individual departments? Usually it is just assigned on the basis of some percentage of budgeted expenses: if a hospital budgets $5 million in expenses and determines that $500,000 profit is required, each department might set its rates to recover 10% above its expenses. However, the importance of cost reimbursement and bad debts at the departmental level should be considered.

Discretionary Revenue Budgets

Discretionary revenue may be important, especially for institutions with large endowments. Any good management control system should establish a budget for expected return on endowments. Variations from the expected level should be investigated; changes in investment management may be necessary.

Capital Budget

Capital budgeting can give many health care managers a major control tool. It can significantly affect the level of cost. This is especially true when not only the initial capital costs associated with given capital expenditures, but associated operating costs for salaries and supplies, are considered. We will discuss the capital budgeting process in more detail in the next chapter.

The Cash Budget

The cash budget is management's best indicator of the organization's expected short-run solvency. It translates all of the above budgets into a statement of cash inflows and outflows. The cash budget is usually broken down by periods within the total budget period, such as months or quarters. Exhibit 6-8 presents an example of a cash budget.

A series of departmental expense budgets, departmental revenue budgets, a discretionary revenue budget and a capital budget that do not provide a sufficient cash flow can necessitate major revisions. If the organization cannot or will not finance these deficits, changes must be made in the budgets to maintain the solvency of the institution. A poor cash budget could cause an increase in rates, a reduction in expenses, a reduction in capital expenditures, or many other changes. These changes and revisions must be made until the cash budget reflects a position of short-run solvency.

Budgeted Financial Statements

The two major financial statements that are developed on a budgetary basis are the balance sheet and the statement of revenues and expenses. These two statements are indicators of both short- and long-run solvency, however they are more important in assessing long-run solvency. Unfavorable projections in either statement might also cause changes in any of the other budgets.

In summary, the budgeted financial statements and the cash budgets test the adequacy of the entire budgetary process. Budgets that result in an unfavorable financial position, as reflected by these three budgets, must be adjusted. Solvency is a goal in most organizations that cannot be sacrificed.

ZERO BASE BUDGETING

Zero base budgeting is a term that has recently gained publicity. It has been touted as management's most effective cost containment tool. It has also been described as the biggest hoax of the century. The truth lies somewhere in the middle.

Zero base budgeting or zero base review, as some like to call it, is a way of looking at existing programs. It is part of programming, but it focuses on existing programs instead of new programs. Zero base budgeting assumes that no existing program is entitled to automatic approval. Many individuals have compared this process with existing budgetary systems that appear to be based on prior year expenditure levels. Zero base budgeting looks at the entire budget and determines the efficacy of the entire expenditure.

The zero base budgeting concept requires a tremendous effort and investment of time. It cannot be done well on an annual basis. This is why many refer to it as zero base review, instead of zero base budgeting. Some individuals have suggested that a zero base review of a given activity would be appropriate every five years.

Zero base budgeting or zero base review refers to a process of periodically reevaluating all the programs and their associated levels of expenditures. Management decides the frequency of this reevaluation and may vary it from every year to every five years.

While most decision makers agree with the concept of zero base budgeting, two significant questions remain unanswered.

- What is the arithmetic used in zero base budgeting?
- Who is involved in the actual decision-making process?

Both questions are important in the success or failure of a zero base budget program. There is not total agreement among experts on these two questions. We will present what we believe to be the basis of the zero base budgeting concept in terms of these two questions. We will illustrate our discussion with an example of an actual application of these principles in the data processing department of a hospital. In this specific example, significant savings were realized through the application of these principles.

The Arithmetic of Zero Base Budgeting

Nearly everyone would agree that cost benefit analysis is the arithmetic of zero base budgeting. There are two important issues in the application of cost benefit analysis in zero base budgeting programs.

1. Are the services presently provided being delivered in an efficient manner?
2. Are the services presently provided being delivered in an effective manner in terms of the organization's goals and objectives?

A framework for quantitatively answering these two questions is important; there are seven sequential steps that must be conducted.

1. Define the outputs or services provided by the program/departmental area.
2. Determine what the costs of these services or outputs are.
3. Identify options for reducing the cost through changes in outputs or services.
4. Identify options for producing the services and outputs more efficiently.
5. Determine the cost savings associated with options identified in steps 3 and 4.
6. Assess the risks, both qualitative and quantitative, associated with the identified options of steps 3 and 4.
7. Select and implement those options with an acceptable cost/risk relationship.

Definition of Outputs

Exhibit 6-9 lists outputs provided by the Data Processing Department. In this case, Data Processing identifies six basic functions or service areas:

1. Outpatient Systems
2. Inpatient Systems
3. Step-Down
4. Month-End
5. Accounts Payable
6. Payroll

Determining the specific outputs of each of these areas as in Exhibit 6-9, is in general a useful procedure. Determining the basic factors behind each department's or program's existence is a good first step in defining specific outputs.

Determination of Costs

The concept of cost that is most relevant is *avoidable cost*. An attempt is made to discover what the costs of these services are now and what cost would be incurred if these services were discontinued. In this context, the direct cost of the department is most useful. Indirect cost in most situations should be ignored because it is unavoidable. In the data processing case the three direct cost components were supplies, labor and machine cost and other. Of these three elements, only labor and machine cost and supply cost are elements which can be avoided, given a reduction in services.

The average supply cost per page was derived by dividing total supply cost less supply cost that could be specifically traced to a specific report by the total number of pages less pages associated with reports for which supply cost could be directly traced:

$$\text{Supply Cost/Page} = \frac{\$24,702 - \$15,065}{1,077,885 - 225,044} = \$.0113$$

The six reports for which supply cost was directly traceable were:

	SYSTEM
• Self-Pay Patient Statement	I-L
• Summary Patient Statement	II-Q
• Detail Patient Statement	II-R
• Time Cards	VI-I
• Standard Payroll Checks	VI-J
• Prepaid Checks	VI-K(1)

Labor and machine cost was divided by weighted pages to determine a cost per weighted page. Weighted pages is an index that attempts to reflect the fact that little or no additional labor and machine cost is incurred for multiple copies of reports. The index uses a base report of two copies to provide the conversion. Thus, a four-copy report consisting of three pages would require twelve total pages, but would be stated as a six-page report when expressed in weighted pages. In certain situations this rule is modified to reflect a more realistic assessment of cost variation. In this department the labor and machine cost per weighted page was

$$\text{Labor \& Machine Cost/Weighted Page} = \frac{\$225,367}{778,900} = \$.2894$$

Options for changes in output

Exhibit 6-10 identifies 11 options for modifying the output of the data processing department. Typical output changes could occur through elimination of the service; reduction in the frequency of the service; reduction in the quality of service; or reduction in the amount of service. All of these specific types of changes, except reduction in quality, occurred in the data processing example.

Options for producing services more efficiently

Only after some idea of the need for services is determined can efficiency be seriously examined. In this example, there are no efficiency options identified. The identification of improved ways to provide services is an important activity in efforts to minimize costs. In a complete zero base review, efficiency should be considered.

Determination of Cost Savings

Exhibit 6-10 identifies the cost savings associated with the output change options identified for the data processing department. Avoidable cost is the cost concept used. The savings are limited to just supply costs when a report is not discontinued, but only the number of copies is changed. When a report is discontinued or its frequency is reduced, then labor and machine costs are also reflected in the savings to be realized. Some may question whether or not actual labor and machine savings could be realized in changes this small. Recognizing that many costs of this type are step or semifixed, the actual incremental cost associated with a very slight reduction in volume may be negligible. However in reviews of this type, where significant changes in work effort are envisioned, the average cost estimate may be a reasonable expectation of savings. In this example, total cost savings from the identified 11 options is projected to be approximately $90,000.

Risk Assessment

Risk is a function of two factors: the probability of an adverse consequence and the potential severity of that consequence. In most situations, both these factors are highly subjective. However, some idea of risk, even subjectively determined, is necessary in the overall assessment of the option's desirability.

Decision Making

After the conclusion of this analysis, someone needs to make a decision concerning which specific options should be selected. This designation falls to those involved in the zero base review or the management structure.

Management Structure

However, there are three major factors that should be considered regarding the management structure to be used in conducting a zero based budget program:

1. For general service or indirect departments, panels of managers from using departments should be involved in identifying options for changes in outputs. These individuals have an interest and a need to know what changes are likely to be made. In addition, their assessment of risk is important.

2. Individuals from the specific program area under evaluation should be involved in the zero base review. Their involvement is essential for two reasons: (1) in many cases, the best ideas for changes in output or changes in methods of production will come from individuals intimately involved in the delivery of those services; (2) participation of these individuals in the review process is more likely to insure cooperation in any decisions that are actually made.

3. Decisions on options should be made by top management. Placing responsibility in lower level management may create problems of suboptimization. Top management needs to make the decisions because they have a total perspective of the organization.

SUMMARY

This chapter has examined budgeting and the management control process. It focused specifically on budgeting and management control as practiced at the institutional or organizational level. Specifically, the control unit under discussion was usually a department. However, the application of the principles of management control discussed in this chapter is much broader. It is possible to think of a control unit as an entire hospital or region, and the controller as a health systems agency or a rate setting organization. Even on this broad scale, the general principles of management control and budgeting should be applicable.

Exhibit 6-1 Hospital Organization Chart

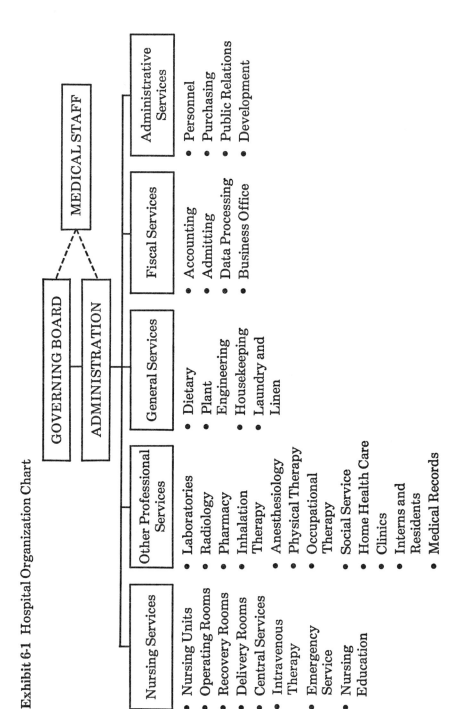

Exhibit 6-2 Management Control Process

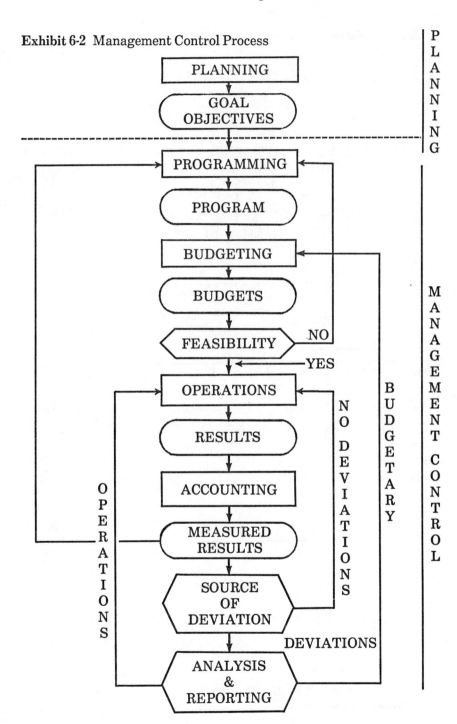

Exhibit 6-3 Integration of the Budgetary Process

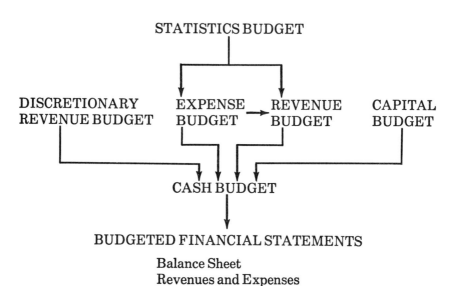

Exhibit 6-4 Laboratory Productivity Data

		1977 Actual	1978
	Hours Worked	Relative Value Units (RVU)	RVUs
January	2,825	5,700	6,270
February	2,700	5,200	5,720
March	2,900	6,000	6,600
April	2,875	5,900	6,490
May	2,825	5,700	6,270
June	2,700	5,200	5,720
July	2,750	5,400	5,940
August	2,625	4,900	5,390
September	2,725	5,300	5,830
October	2,750	5,400	5,940
November	2,750	5,400	5,940
December	2,775	5,500	6,050
TOTAL	33,200	65,600	72,160

$$1977 \text{ Average Hours/RVU} = \frac{33,200}{65,600} = .5061$$

Exhibit 6-5 Alternative Hours Worked Budget for Laboratory

	Forecast Budget*	Flexible Budget**
January	3,043	2,967
February	3,043	2,830
March	3,043	3,050
April	3,043	3,022
May	3,043	2,967
June	3,043	2,830
July	3,043	2,885
August	3,043	2,747
September	3,043	2,857
October	3,043	2,885
November	3,043	2,885
December	3,043	2,912
TOTAL	36,516	34,837

*$(.5061 \times 72,160)/12 = 3043.35$
**January Value $= (1,400) + (.25 \times 6270)$

Exhibit 6-6 Standard Cost Variance Analysis for Labor Costs
Laboratory, January 1978

1. Price Variance = (Actual Hours Worked × Actual Wage Rate)
   − (Actual Hours Worked × Budgeted Wage Rate)
   $= (3,100 \times \$10.00) - (3,100 \times \$9.00) = \$3100$
   [Unfavorable]

2. Efficiency Variance = (Actual Hours Worked
   × Budgeted Wage Rate)
   − (Budgeted Hours Worked
   × Budgeted Wage Rate) $= (3,100 \times \$9.00)$
   $- (3,025 \times \$9.00) = \$675$ [Unfavorable]

3. Total Variance $= \$3,100 + \$675 = \$3,775$ [Unfavorable]

Actual Wage Rate $= \$31,000/3,100 = \$10.00$
Budgeted Wage Rate $= \$9.00$
Actual Hours Worked $= 3,100$
Budgeted Hours Worked $= (1,400) + (.25 \times 6,500) = 3,025$

Exhibit 6-7 Rate Setting in the Revenue Budget

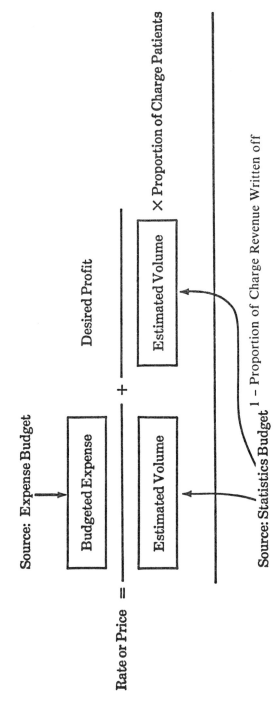

Note: The two source items indicate where values for budgeted expense and estimated volume may be found.

Exhibit 6-8 Cash Budget, Budget Year 1978

| | 1st Quarter | | | | | |
	January	February	March	2nd Quarter	3rd Quarter	4th Quarter
Receipts from Operations	$300,000	$310,000	$320,000	$1,000,000	$1,100,000	$1,100,000
Disbursements from Operations	280,000	280,000	300,000	940,000	1,000,000	1,000,000
Cash Available from Operations	$ 20,000	$ 30,000	$ 20,000	$ 60,000	$ 100,000	$ 100,000
Other Receipts						
Increase in Mortgage Payable				500,000		
Sale of Fixed Assets		20,000				
Unrestricted Income-Endowment			40,000	40,000	40,000	40,000
Total Other Receipts	–0–	$ 20,000	$ 40,000	$ 540,000	$ 40,000	$ 40,000
Other Disbursements						
Mortgage Payments						
Fixed Asset Purchase			150,000	480,000	150,000	
Funded Depreciation			130,000	130,000	30,000	30,000

Exhibit 6-8 continued

| | 1st Quarter | | | | | |
	January	February	March	2nd Quarter	3rd Quarter	4th Quarter
Total Other Disbursement	-0-	-0-	180,000	510,000	180,000	30,000
Net Cash Gain (loss)	$ 20,000	$ 50,000	$(120,000)	90,000	(40,000)	110,000
Beginning Cash Balance	100,000	120,000	170,000	50,000	140,000	100,000
Cumulative Cash	$120,000	$170,000	$ 50,000	$ 140,000	$ 100,000	$ 210,000
Desired Level of Cash	100,000	100,000	100,000	100,000	100,000	100,000
Cash Above Minimum Needs (Financing Needs)	$ 20,000	$ 70,000	$(50,000)	$ 40,000	-0-	$ 110,000

Exhibit 6-9 Data Processing Outputs and Costs

	Pages	Runs Per Year	Copies	Total Pages	Weighted Pages	$.0113/pg. Direct Supply Cost	$.2894/wtd. pg. cost Labor&Mach.	Total Cost	Cost Reductions
I. OUTPATIENT SYSTEM									
A. Outpatient Maintenance Report	2	365	4	2,920	1,460	$33.00	$422.49	$455.49	($8.25)
B. Outpatient Error Listing for Admissions	2	365	4	2,920	1,460	33.00	422.49	455.49	(8.25)
C. Outpatient Initial Edit Summary	1	365	4	1,460	730	16.50	211.24	227.74	(4.13)
1. Admissions Summary Total	1	365	4	1,460	730	16.50	211.24	227.74	(4.13)
2. Initial Cash Edit	1								
3. Additional Patients Added to Outpatient History		365	4	1,460	730	16.50	211.24	227.74	(4.13)
D. Daily Transaction Audit Report—Charges	11	365	4	16,060	8,030	181.48	2,323,69	2505.17	(45.37)
E. Outpatient Posting Control	40	365	4	58,400	29,200	659.92	8,449.78	9,189.70	(164.95)
F. Daily Revenue Report	42	365	4	61,320	30,660	692.92	8,872.27	9,565.19	(9,565.19)

Exhibit 6-9 continued

	Pages	Runs Per Year	Copies	Total Pages	Weighted Pages	$.0113/pg. Direct Supply Cost	$.2894/wtd. pg. cost Labor&Mach.	Total Cost	Cost Reductions
G. Outpatient Billing Balance	4	365	4	5,840	2,920	65.99	844.98	910.27	(16.50)
H. Patients Transferred to AR/History File	5	365	4	7,300	3,650	82.49	1,056.22	1,138.71	(20.62)
I. Cash Receipts and Adjustments Report	3	365	4	4,380	2,190	49.49	633.73	683.22	(12.37)
J. AR Transaction Audit	5	365	4	7,300	3,650	82.49	1,056.22	1,138.71	(20.62)
K. AR Error Listing	4	365	4	1,460	730	16.50	211.24	227.74	(4.13)
L. Self-Pay Patient Statement*	100	365	1	36,500	36,500	3,650.00	10,562.22	14,212.22	
M. Revenue and Usage Statistics	42	365	2	30,660	30,660	346.46	8,872.27	9,218.73	
N. General Journal	3	12	2	72	72	81	20.84	21.65	
O. Outpatient Edit Report	5	12	2	120	120	1.36	34.73	36.09	
P. Outpatient Activity Trial Balance	2,500	12	2	60,000	60,000	678.00	17,362.56	18,040.56	
Q. Outpatient Alpha Listing (Telephone)	800	52	4	166,400	83,200	1,880.32	24,076.08	25,906.00	(25,956.40)
R. Outpatient Alpha Listing (Balance)	800	52	4	166,400	83,200	1,880.32	24,076.08	25,956.40	(25,956.40)

Exhibit 6-9 continued

	Pages	Runs Per Year	Copies	Total Pages	Weighted Pages	$.0113/pg. Direct Supply Cost	$.2894/wtd. pg. cost Labor&Mach.	Total Cost	Cost Reductions
II. INPATIENT SYSTEM									
A. Final Census Report	27	365	4	39,420	19,710	$ 445.45	$5,703.60	$6,149.05	($222.75)
B. Volunteer Alpha Listing	6	365	3	6,570	4,380	74.24	1,267.47	1,341.71	
C. Alphabetic Census	6	365	6	13,140	4,380	148.48	1,267.47	1,415.95	
D. Financial Class Census Report	10	365	2	7,300	7,300	82.49	2,112.44	2,194.93	(2,194.93)
E. Utilization Census	6	365	4	8,760	4,380	98.99	1,267.47	1,366.46	(50.00)
F. Social Services Census	10	365	1	3,650	7,300	41.25	2,112.44	2,153.69	
G. Statistical Census Reports	2	365	3	2,190	1,460	24.75	422.49	447.24	(447.24)
H. Clergy Listing	15	365	1	5,475	10,950	61.87	3,168.69	3,230.54	
I. Admission, Discharge and Transfer Report	4	365	8	11,680	2,920	131.98	844.98	976.96	
J. Pap Smear Admissions Control Report	1	365	2	730	730	8.25	211.24	219.49	
K. Census by H-ICDA Code	7	365	2	5,110	5,110	57.74	1,478.71	1,536.45	
L. Daily Charge Transaction Error Listing	5	365	1	1,825	3,650	20.62	1,056.22	1,076.84	

Exhibit 6-9 continued

	Pages	Runs Per Year	Copies	Total Pages	Weighted Pages	$.0113/pg. Direct Supply Cost	$.2894/wtd. pg. cost Labor&Mach.	Total Cost	Cost Reductions
M. Daily Transaction	44	365	1	16,060	32,120	181.48	9,294.76	9,476.24	
N. Daily Dialysis Report	1	365	2	730	730	8.25	211.24	219.49	
O. Inpatient Billing Balance	8	365	2	5,840	5,840	65.99	1,689.96	1,755.95	
P. Outpatient Billing Balance—Dialysis	2	365	2	1,460	1,460	16.50	422.49	438.99	
Q. Summary Patient Statement*	50	365	2	36,500	36,500	1,825.00	10,562.22	12,387.22	
R. Detail Patient Statement*	50	365	2	36,500	36,500	1,825.00	10,562.22	12,387.22	
S. Noncovered Charges	10	365	1	3,650	7,300	41.25	2,112.44	2,153.69	
T. New Accounts Receivable Report	3	365	2	2,190	2,190	24.75	633.73	658.48	
U. Cash Receipts and Adjustments	10	365	3	10,950	7,300	123.74	2,112.44	2,236.18	
V. AR Transaction Audit	10	365	2	7,300	7,300	82.49	2,112.44	2,194.93	
W. Daily Error Listing	3	365	2	2,190	2,190	24.75	633.73	658.48	
X. Schedule of PreAdmission	3	365	2	2,190	2,190	24.75	633.73	658.48	
Y. Medicaid Review Census	2	365	2	1,460	1,460	16.50	422.49	438.99	

Exhibit 6-9 continued

	Pages	Runs Per Year	Copies	Total Pages	Weighted Pages	$.0113/pg. Direct Supply Cost	$.2894/wtd. pg. cost Labor&Mach.	Total Cost	Cost Reductions
III. STEP DOWN									
A. Step Down Cost Center Description Table	2	12	2	48	48				
B. Step Down Allocations Master File	2	12	2	48	48	$ .54	$ 13.89	$ 14.93	
C. Step Down Direct Expense Edit	2	12	2	48	48	.54	13.89	14.43	
D. Step Down Cost Allocation Statistics File	2	12	2	48	48	.54	13.89	14.93	
E. Step Down Cost Allocation—Periodic	2	12	2	48	48	.54	13.89	14.93	
IV. MONTH END									
A. Cummulative Monthly Statistical Census	1	12	2	24	24	.27	6.95	7.22	
B. Monthly Statistical Census by Day	1	12	2	24	24	.27	6.95	7.22	
C. Infection Control Report	1	12	2	24	24	.27	6.95	7.22	

Exhibit 6-9 continued

	Pages	Runs Per Year	Copies	Total Pages	Weighted Pages	$.0113/pg. Direct Supply Cost	$.2894/wtd. pg. cost Labor&Mach.	Total Cost	Cost Reductions
D. Reimbursement Summary	1	12	2	24	24	.27	6.95	7.22	
E. Revenue and Usage Statistics	65	12	2	1,560	1,560	17.63	451.43	469.06	
F. Aged Accounts Receivable Summary	1	12	2	24	24	.27	6.95	7.22	
G. Detail Trial Balance	105	12	2	2,520	2,520	28.48	729.22	757.70	
H. In-House 21 Days Billing	25	12	2	600	600	6.78	173.63	180.41	
I. Dialysis Billing	89	12	2	2,136	2,136	24.14	618.11	642.25	
J. Zero Balance Roster	742	12	4	35,616	17,808	402.46	5,153.21	5,555.67	($5555.67)
K. Bad Debt Report	35	12	2	840	840	9.49	243.08	252.57	
L. General Journal	5	12	2	120	120	1.36	34.73	36.09	
V. ACCOUNTS PAYABLE SYSTEM									
A. Vendor Master Maintenance Report	2	156	2	624	624	7.05	180.57	187.62	
B. AP Initial Edit Listing	1	156	2	312	312	3.53	90.29	93.82	

Exhibit 6-9 continued

	Pages	Runs Per Year	Copies	Total Pages	Weighted Pages	$.0113/pg. Direct Supply Cost	$.2894/wtd. pg. cost Labor&Mach.	Total Cost	Cost Reductions
C. AP Batch Proof	1	156	2	312	312	3.53	90.29	93.82	
D. Cash Requirements Report	50	12	2	1,200	1,200	13.56	347.25	360.81	
E. AP Monthly Reconciliation	30	12	2	720	720	8.14	208.35	216.49	
F. AP Distribution	23	12	2	552	552	6.24	159.74	165.98	
G. AP Trial Balance	50	12	2	1,200	1,200	13.56	347.25	360.81	
H. Vendor Master Listing	2	12	2	48	48	.54	13.89	14.43	
VI. PAYROLL									
A. Payroll Edit Summary									
1. Payroll Update Controls	1	104	2	208	208	$ 2.35	$ 60.19	$ 62.54	
2. Payroll Master File Maintenance	10	104	2	2,080	2,080	23.50	601.90	625.40	
B. Time Card Edit Report	60	52	4	12,480	6,240	141.02	1,805.71	1,946.73	
C. Check Register	58	52	2	6,032	6,032	68.16	1,745.52	1,813.68	
D. Department Benefits Statement	60	52	4	12,480	6,240	141.02	1,805.71	1,946.73	
E. Labor Analysis Report	42	52	2	4,368	4,368	49.36	1,263.99	1,313.35	

Exhibit 6-9 continued

	Pages	Runs Per Year	Copies	Total Pages	Weighted Pages	$.0113/pg. Direct Supply Cost	$.2894/wtd. pg. cost Labor&Mach.	Total Cost	Cost Reductions
F. Payroll Journal Report	10	12	1	120	240	1.36	69.45	70.81	
G. Quarterly 941 Report	27	4	2	216	216	2.44	62.51	64.95	
H. W-2 Forms	1,091	1	1	1,091	2,182	12.33	631.42	643.75	
I. Time Cards*	1,091	52	1	56,732	56,732	4,252.50	16,416.88	20,669.38	($10,334.69)
J. Standard Payroll Checks*	1,091	52	1	56,732	56,732	3,373.65	16,416.88	19,710.53	(9,855.26)
K. Miscellaneous Reports									
1. Employee Longevity Report	10	12	2	240	240	2.70	69.45	72.15	
2. YTD Earnings Report	1,091	4	2	8,728	8,728	98.68	2,525.67	2,524.29	
3. Union Dues Paid	8	12	2	192	192	2.17	55.56	57.73	
4. Estimated Yearly Budget Report by Status and by Grade	60	1	1	60	120	68	34.73	35.41	
5. Sick Hour Control Report (not done)									

Exhibit 6-9 continued

	Pages	Runs Per Year	Copies	Total Pages	Weighted Pages	$.0113/pg. Direct Supply Cost	$.2894/wtd. pg. cost Labor&Mach.	Total Cost	Cost Reductions
6. Prepaid Checks	20	104	1	2,080	2,080	138.76	601.90	740.66	
7. LPN Listing	2	2	2	8	8	.09	2.31	2.40	
8. Employee Address Labels (30/page)	30	2	1	60	60	.68	17.17	17.85	
9. Century Club Membership Labels* (not done)									
				1,077,885	778,900	$24,702.00	$225,367.00	$250,069.00	($90,138.00)

*Items for which supplies were directly costed.
Total pages for these items were 225,044 and total direct supply cost was $15,065.

Exhibit 6-10 Options for Reducing Output in Data Processing
Department

Option	Risk	Savings
1. Reduce outpatient report copies I-A-K from four copies to three copies per day.	small	$ 314.48
2. Change usage demand on outpatient report I-F from daily to monthly.	small	9,251.02
3. Eliminate two copies of inpatient report II-A—final census.	small	222.75
4. Discontinue inpatient report II-D— financial class census.	small	2,194.93
5. Eliminate two copies of inpatient report I-E—utilization census.	small	50.00
6. Eliminate outpatient report I-Q—alpha listing with telephone number.	small	25,956.40
7. Eliminate outpatient report I-R—alpha listing with balance.	small	25,956.40
8. Eliminate inpatient report II-G— statistical census.	small	447.24
9. Eliminate zero balance roster report— month end—report II-J	small	5,555.67
10. Pay bi-weekly rather than weekly; cut preparation and usage of time cards by 50%.	medium	10,334.69
11. Pay bi-weekly rather than weekly; reduce paychecks preparation and usage by 50%.	medium	9,855.26
TOTAL ESTIMATED SAVINGS		90,137.84

Chapter 7

Capital Project Analysis

The topic of this final chapter is capital project analysis, which is broadly defined to include two major aspects of decision making:

- selection of investment projects
- selection of sources of financing

Capital project analysis falls in the programming phase of the management control process. While zero base budgeting or zero base review can be thought of as the programming phase of management control concerned with old or existing programs, capital project analysis is the phase primarily concerned with new programs. It is an ongoing activity, but is not usually summarized annually in the budget. The capital budget is the yearly estimate of resources that will be expended for new programs during the coming year. Capital budgeting may be thought of as less comprehensive and shorter-term than capital project analysis.

PARTIES INVOLVED

The capital decision-making process in the health care industry is complex for several reasons. First, the stated goals and objectives of a health care facility are likely to be more complex and less quantifiable than those of a for-profit firm where profit is the major, if not exclusive, goal. Second, the number of individuals involved in the process, either directly or indirectly, is likely to be greater in the health care industry than in most other industries. Exhibit 7-1 illustrates the relationships of various parties involved in the capital decision-making process of a health care facility.

External Parties

Financing Sources

The availability of external funding for many new programs is an important variable in the capital decision-making process. There are a variety of individual organizations involved in the credit determination process, including investment bankers, bond rating agencies, bankers and feasibility consultants. Many of these organizations and their roles will be discussed later in this chapter. At the present time, it is important to recognize that collectively, these parties may influence the amount of money which can be borrowed and the terms of the borrowing. These decisions affect the nature and size of capital projects which may be undertaken by any given health care facility.

Rate Setting and Rate Control Agencies

Many states have agencies that set and control the rates hospitals and other health care facilities can charge for services. In addition the federal government, during the Economic Stabilization Program 1971-1974, established a nationwide system of rate review and control which could be reenacted at any given point in time. The nature of influence exerted by rate setting or rate control organizations on capital decision making is indirect but extremely important. Control of rates can limit both short-term and long-term profitability. This control can reduce a health care facility's ability to repay indebtedness and thus limit its access to the capital markets. More directly, rate setting organizations can limit the amount of money available for financing capital projects by reducing the amount of profits that may be retained. One of the major effects of rate control in the economic stabilization program era was a significant reduction in the level of capital expenditures by hospitals.

Third Party Payers

Like rate setting and rate control agencies, third party payers can influence the capital decision-making process indirectly. Through their reimbursement provisions, both capital expenditure levels and sources of financing may be affected. For example, many individuals feel that third party cost reimbursement provides a strong incentive for increased capital spending: in most situations, cost reimbursement provides for the reimbursement of depreciation and interest expense, which may then be used to repay financial requirements associated with any indebtedness. As a result, the risk associated with hospital indebtedness is reduced. This has favorably affected the availability of credit and the terms associated with that credit in the hospital industry.

Planning Agencies

Because of the provisions contained in Public Laws 92-603 and 93-641, health systems agencies directly influence the capital expenditure decision-making process of health care facilities who receive federal monies from Title V (Maternal and Child Health), XVIII (Medicare), or XIX (Medicaid) of the Social Security Act. In many situations, these agencies can permit or deny approval of a capital expenditure, although the state designated planning agency technically has such authority. Exhibit 7-2 provides a schematic representation of the review process that exists under Section 1122 of the Social Security Act.

Internal Parties

Board of Trustees

Ultimately the Board of Trustees is responsible for the capital expenditure and capital financing program of any given health care facility. However, in most normal situations the board delegates this authority to management and special board committees. The board's major function should be to establish clearly defined goals and objectives. The statement of goals and objectives is a prerequisite to the programming phase of management control which comprises capital expenditure analysis. Without a clear statement capital expenditure programs cannot be adequately defined and analyzed.

Planning Committee

Many health care facility boards of trustees have established planning committees whose primary function is to define, analyze and propose programs that may help the organization attain its goals and objectives. They are specialized groups, within the board of trustees, that are directly involved in capital expenditure analysis.

Finance Committee

Some boards of trustees have also established a finance committee which has authority for several key financial functions, including budgeting and capital financing. Both are involved with translating programs, perhaps identified by the planning committee, into financing requirements. These requirements may be operational or capital. Insuring a supply of financing to meet these program requirements is the financial committee's major objective. Many of its budgetary functions are delegated to the controller, many of its capital financing functions to the treasurer.

Administration

The administration is responsible on a day-to-day basis for implementing approved capital expenditure programs and developing related financing plans. The administration must develop an organizational system that responds to departmental managers' and medical staff's requests for capital expenditures. Much of the authority that is vested in the administrator's position is delegated by the board of trustees. In addition, the administration may also seek board approval for its own programs.

Departmental Managers

Departmental managers make most internal requests for capital expenditure approval. In many health care facilities, formal systems for approving capital expenditures are developed to receive, process and answer the requests. Allocating a limited capital budget to competing departmental areas is a difficult task for management. Carefully defining criteria for capital decision making can help make this problem less political and more objective.

Medical Staff

Medical staff demands for capital expenditures are a problem unique to the health care industry. Medical staff members, in most situations, are not employees of the health care facility but use it to treat their private patients. Because of their ability to change a facility's use patterns dramatically and thus affect financial solvency, administrators listen to, and frequently honor, their wishes. Health care facilities are thus faced with strong pressure from individuals who have little financial interest in their organization, whose financial interest may in fact oppose the organization's.

Controller

The controller's function in many small health care facilities may be merged with the treasurer's. However, the controller notably facilitates capital expenditure approval. The controller is usually responsible for developing capital expenditure request forms, and for assisting departmental managers in preparing their capital expenditure proposals. The controller usually serves as an analyst, assisting the administrator in allocating the budget to competing departmental areas.

Treasurer

The treasurer is responsible for obtaining funds both in the short and long run. The treasurer may work in relation with the financial committee to negotiate for funds necessary to implement approved programs.

CLASSIFICATION OF CAPITAL EXPENDITURES

A capital expenditure is a commitment of resources that is expected to provide benefits over a reasonably long period of time, at least two or more years. Any system of management control needs to consider the types of capital expenditure. Different types raise different problems; they may require specific individuals to evaluate them, or special methods of evaluation.

Several of the more important classifications of capital expenditures to be considered are—

- time period over which the investment occurs
- type of resources invested
- dollar amount of capital expenditures
- type of benefits received

Time Period of Investment

Determining the amount of resources committed to a capital project depends heavily upon the definition of the time period. For example, how would you determine the capital expenditures needed by a project which had a very low initial investment cost, but a significant investment cost in future years? Should just the initial capital expenditure be considered, or should total expenditures over the life of the project be considered too? If the latter is the answer, is it appropriate just to add the total expenditures together, or should expenditures made in later years be weighted to reflect their lower present value? If so, at what discount rate? These are not simple questions to answer, but they are very important in evaluating capital projects.

A classic example of this type of problem in the health care industry is the initiation of programs that have been funded by grants. In many situations, there appears to be little or no investment of capital expenditure since the amounts are funded almost totally through a grant. Projects thus appear to be highly desirable. However, if there is a formal or informal commitment to continue programs for a longer period of time, capital expenditures and additional operating funds for later periods may be required. It is imperative that grant funded projects be classified separately and their long-run capital cost requirements identified. The health care facility may very well not have a sufficient capital base to finance a program's continuation. Granting agencies should also assess health care facilities' financial capability to continue funded programs after the grant period expires.

Type of Resources Invested

When discussing capital expenditures, many individuals are apt to limit their attention to just the expenditure or resources invested in capital assets, that is tangible fixed assets. This consideration has several shortcomings and may result in ineffective capital expenditure decisions.

First, focusing on tangible fixed assets implies ownership, yet many health care facilities *lease* a significant percentage of their fixed assets, especially in the major movable equipment area. If a lease is not construed to be a capital expenditure, it may escape the normal review and approval system, for *both* the internal review and approval process and the review and approval process of a health systems agency. Lease payments should be considered as a capital expenditure. Furthermore, the contractual provisions of the lease should be considered in determining the total expenditure amount. Weight should be given to future payments or to the alternative purchase price of the asset.

Second, the capital costs of a capital expenditure are only one part of total cost: in the labor intensive health care industry, these capital costs may be just the tip of the iceberg. All of the operating costs associated with beginning and continuing a capital project should be considered. Programs with very low capital investment costs may not look as good when their operating costs are considered.

Life cycle costing is a method for estimating the cost of capital projects which reflects total costs, both operating and capital, and reflects those costs over the project's estimated useful life. The life cycle cost of all contemplated programs should be considered—failure can cause errors in the capital decision-making process, especially in the selection of alternative programs. Consider two alternative renal dialysis projects: both may have the same capacity, but one may have a significantly greater investment cost because it uses equipment requiring less monitoring and lower operating costs. Failure to consider the operating cost differences between these two projects may bias the decision in favor of the project with lower capital expenditures, and result in higher expenses in the long run.

Amount of the Expenditure

Different systems of control and evaluation are required for different sized projects. It would not be economical to spend $500 in administrative time evaluating the purchase of a $100 calculator. Nor would it be wise to spend only $500 to evaluate a $25 million building program. Obviously control over capital expenditures should be conditioned by the total amount involved, and if appropriate, the amount should be based on the total life cycle cost.

Controlling capital expenditures in most organizations, including health care facilities, typically follows one of three patterns:

1. approval required for all dollar size capital expenditures;
2. approval required for all dollar size capital expenditures above a preestablished limit; or
3. no approval required for individual capital expenditure projects below a total budgeted amount for the responsibility center.

Retaining final approval of all capital expenditures lets management exert maximum control over this resource spending area. However, the cost of management time to develop and review these proposals is high. In most organizations of any size, management review of all ·capital expenditure requests is not productive. However, some review is needed, so a limit may be established. For example, a given responsibility center or department may not submit any justification for individual capital expenditure projects requiring less than $200 in investment cost. In such a case, there is usually some formal or informal limitation on the total dollar size of the capital budget that will be available for small dollar capital expenditures. This prevents responsibility center managers from making excessive investments in capital expenditures that have no formalized reviewing system.

Another form of management control over capital expenditures is an absolute dollar limit: any responsibility center manager may spend up to an authorized capital budget on any items in question. The real negotiation involves determining the size of the capital budget that will be available for individual departments. This system, while least costly in terms of review time, does not insure that the capital expenditures actually made are necessarily in the best interests of the organization.

Types of Benefits

Depending upon the types of benefits envisioned for a capital expenditure, different systems of management control and evaluation may be necessary. For example, investment in a medical office building brings different benefits than investment in an alcoholic rehabilitation unit. Such differences make it inappropriate to rely exclusively on any one method of evaluating projects. This is important: *traditional methods of evaluating capital budgeting may not be appropriate in the health care industry.* Traditional methods evaluate only the financial aspects of a capital expenditure. Projects in the health care industry may produce benefits that are far more important than a reduction in cost or an increase in profit.

Major types of benefits which affect the method of evaluation to be considered are:

- operational continuance
- financial
- other

The first category of investments produces benefits that permit continuance of operations of the facility along its present lines. The governing board or management must usually make two decisions. (1) Are continued operations in the present form desirable? In most cases the answer is affirmative. (2) Which alternative investment project can achieve continued operations in the most desirable way (e.g. lowest cost, patient safety, etc.)? A classic example of this type of investment is a licensure requirement for installation of a sprinkler system in a nursing home. Failure to make the investment may imply discontinuance of operations.

The second category of investment provides benefits that are largely financial, either reduced cost or increased profits to the organization. Many individuals may initially believe that these two are identical, that reduced costs imply increased profits. However, as we will see, this may not be true in the cost reimbursement world in which most health care facilities operate. The important point to remember is that since the major benefits are financial, then traditional capital budgeting methods may be more appropriate.

The third category of investments is a catch-all category. It would range from projects that activate major, new medical areas like outpatient or mental health services to projects that improve employee working conditions like employee gymnasiums. Benefits may be harder to quantify and evaluate here. Traditional capital budgeting methods may thus be appropriate only in the selection of least costly ways to provide designated services.

THE CAPITAL PROJECT DECISION-MAKING PROCESS

Making decisions on which capital projects will be undertaken is not easy. In many respects it may be the most difficult and important management decision area. The allocation of limited resources to specific project areas will directly affect the efficiency and effectiveness, and ultimately the continued viability, of the organization.

For our purposes we will divide the capital decision-making process into four interrelated activities or stages:

- generation of project information
- evaluation of projects
- decision about which projects to fund
- project implementation and reporting

Generation of Project Information

In this phase of the decision-making process, information is gathered which can later be analyzed and evaluated. It is an extremely important phase because inadequate or inaccurate information can lead to bad decision making. Specifically, there are six major categories of information that should be included in most capital expenditure proposals:

1. alternatives available
2. resources available
3. cost data
4. benefit data
5. prior performance
6. risk projections

Alternatives Available

A major deficiency in many capital expenditure decisions is the failure to consider possible alternatives. Too many times capital expenditures are presented on a take it or leave it basis, but there usually are alternatives. For example, different manufacturers might be selected, different methods of financing could be used, or different boundaries in the scope of the project could be defined.

Resources Available

Capital expenditure decisions are not made in a vacuum. In most situations there are constraints on the amount of available funding.

This is the whole rationale behind capital expenditure decision making: scarce resources must be allocated among a virtually unlimited number of investment opportunities. There is little question about the necessity of information concerning the availability of funding at the top level of management. However, there is some question about its importance at the departmental level. On one hand, a budgetary constraint may temper requests for capital expenditures. On the other hand, it may encourage a departmental manager only to submit those projects that are in the department's best interests. These may, in fact, conflict with the broader goals and objectives of the organization as a whole.

Cost Data

It goes without saying that cost information is an important variable in the decision-making process. The life cycle costs of a project, particularly, should be presented. Limiting cost information just to capital costs can be counterproductive.

Benefit Data

We shall divide benefit data into two categories: quantitative and nonquantitative. There is some feeling that much of the benefit data in the health care industry is nonquantitative. To a large extent, many individuals have seen quantitative data as synonomous with financial data. Since financial criteria are relatively less important in the nonprofit health care industry, the assumption is that quantitative data is also less important. This is not true. Quantitative data can and should be used: effective management control is predicated upon the use of numbers that relate to the organization's stated goals and objectives. It may not be easy to develop quantitative estimates of benefits, but it is not impossible. For example, a hospital in an urban area opens a clinic in a medically underserved area. One of the stated goals for the clinic is the reduction of unnecessary use of the hospital's emergency room for nonurgent care. A realistic and quantifiable benefit of this program should be a numerical reduction in the use of the hospital's emergency room for nonurgent care by individuals from the clinic area. However, no quantitative assessments are either projected or reported; the only quantitative statistics used are those of a financial nature. The management control process in this situation is less valuable than it should have been.

Prior Performance

Information on prior operating results of projects proposed by responsibiltiy center managers can be useful. A comparison of prior, actual results with forecast results can give a decision maker some idea of the manager's reliability in forecasting. In too many cases, project planners are likely to overstate the project's benefits if the project interests them. Review of prior performance can help a manager evaluate the accuracy of the projections. This principle can be applied to the review of projects by health systems agencies.

Risk Projections

Nothing is certain in this world except death and taxes, especially when evaluating capital expenditure projects. It is important to ask "what if" questions. For example, how would costs and benefits change if volume changed? Volume of service is a key variable in most capital expenditure forecasts, and its effects should be understood. In some situations requiring projections for most likely optimistic and pessimistic projections of volume helps answer the questions. The same type of calculations can be made for other key factors, such as prices of key inputs and technological changes. This is an important area to understand because some capital expenditure projects are inherently more risky than others. Specifically, programs with extremely high proportions of fixed or sunk costs are far more sensitive to changes in volume than those with low percentages of fixed or sunk costs.

Evaluation of Projects

While financial criteria are clearly not the only factors that should be evaluated in capital expenditure decisions, there are few, if any, capital expenditure decisions that can omit financial considerations. Our focus is on two of the prime financial criteria: solvency and cost.

Solvency is the first important financial consideration. A project that cannot show a positive rate of return in the long run should be questioned. If implemented, such a program will need to be subsidized by some other existing program area. For example, should a hospital subsidize a outpatient clinic? If so, to what extent? This is the kind of policy and *financial* question the governing board of the organization needs to determine. The fairness of some patients subsidizing other patients is one of the basic qualitative issues in capital project analysis. Furthermore, running an insolvent program can eventually threaten the solvency of the entire organization. Organizations which plan to subsidize insolvent programs must be in good financial condition. Assessing financial condition can only be done after the organization's financial statements are examined.

Cost is the second important financial concern. An organization needs to select the projects that contribute most to the attainment of its objectives, given resource constraints. This type of analysis is often called cost benefit analysis. Benefits differ from project to project. Decision makers evaluating alternative programs must weight those benefits according to their own preferences and compare them to cost.

There is a second dimension to the cost criterion. All projects which are eventually selected should cost the least to provide the service. This type of evaluation is sometimes called cost effectiveness analysis. Least cost should be defined as the present value of both operating and capital costs. Methods for determining this will be discussed later.

Deciding Which Projects to Fund

At this juncture of the capital expenditure decision-making process, it is time to make the decisions. In front of the decision maker(s) is a list of possible projects which may be funded. Each project should represent the lowest cost method of providing the desired service or output. In addition, various benefit data on each project are described. This data should be consistent with the criteria that the decision maker(s) used in their capital expenditure decision making.

To illustrate this process, assume that the governing board is deciding on how many, if any, of three proposed programs it will fund in the coming year, including a burn care unit, a hemodialysis unit and a commercial laboratory. Furthermore, assume that the governing board has decided that there are only four criteria of importance to them:

1. solvency
2. incremental management time required
3. public image
4. medical staff approval

Since no project clearly dominates, it is not obvious which should be funded, if any. Decision makers must weight the criteria according to their own preferences and determine the overall ranking of the three projects. For example, one manager might weight solvency and management time very highly relative to public image and medical staff. He might thus select the commercial laboratory project. Another manager might weight medical staff and public image more heavily and thus select the hemodialysis or burn care unit projects.

The projects have been ranked in terms of their relative attainment of each of these four criteria, as presented below.

PROJECTS

CRITERIA	Hemodialysis Unit	Burn Care Unit	Commercial Laboratory
Solvency	2	3	1
Management Time	2	3	1
Public Image	2	1	3
Medical Staff	1	2	3

Implementation and Reporting Results

Most capital expenditure control systems are concerned primarily, if not exclusively, with analysis and evaluation prior to selection. However, a very real concern—not only in the evaluation of approved projects by institutional managers but in the evaluation of health care facilities and their proposals by health systems agencies—should be whether the projected benefits are actually being realized as forecast. Without this feedback on the actual results of prior investments, the capital expenditure control system has a feedback loop that is not complete. Some of the specific advantages of establishing a capital expenditure review program are listed below.

1. Capital expenditure review could highlight differences in planned versus actual performance that may permit corrective action. If actual performance is never evaluated, corrective action may not be taken. This could mean that the projected benefits might never be realized.

2. Use of a review process may result in more accurate estimates. If individuals realize that they will be held responsible for their estimates, they may tend to be more careful with their projections. This will insure greater accuracy in forecast results.

3. Forecasts by individuals with a continuous record of biased forecasts can be adjusted to reflect that bias. This should result in a better forecast of actual results.

TIME VALUE OF MONEY

In many methods of evaluating both capital expenditure projects and capital financing plans the concept of the time value of money is important. The concept is based on the scarcity of money. Receiving $100 in ten years is not as valuable as receiving $100 in five years, or receiving it right now. In most situations we are interested in the value of money at one of two points in time: (1) the present value, and (2) the future value.

Present Value

Assume that a hospital can lease an asset for $1,000 per year for its four-year estimated life. If the hospital could borrow money at ten percent and buy this asset for $2,800, should it lease or buy?

The answer can be obtained by discounting the lease payment at the hospital borrowing rate of ten percent. Discounting these payments yields the "present value" of the payments. Exhibit 7-3 presents the discount factors that can be used to determine the present value of this stream of lease payments at ten percent:

Year	Discount Factor (@ 10%)	Present Value of $1,000	Year Paid 1	2	3	4
1	.909	$909 ◄————1000			
2	.826	826 ◄————————1000			
3	.751	751 ◄————————————1000			
4	.683	683 ◄————————————————1000			
TOTAL	3.169	$3169				

Several conclusions can be drawn from the above discounting. First, the hospital should purchase the asset rather than lease it, if the borrowing rate is ten percent; the present value cost of the lease is $3,169 which is greater than the $2,800 purchase price. Second, if the payments in each year are equal, which in this case they are, each year's payment does not need to be individually discounted. Instead, the discount factor for each of the individual years can be totalled and that amount multiplied by the yearly payment. In the above example, 3.169 multiplied by $1,000 yields the present value of the lease payments. Exhibit 7-4 gives a table with these values already calculated. Third, all the payments are assumed to be received on the last day of the year. The discount factors are based on one full year of discounting.

Future Value

In other cases, a decision maker may be interested in the future value of a payment or stream of payments at some point in time. Calculating the future value of money payments is often referred to as compounding. For example, assume that an extended care facility wants to set aside $1,000 a year in an account to provide a pool of money for eventual plant and equipment replacement. If the extended care facility can earn ten percent on its investment, what sum of money would it have at the end of four years? Compounding these deposits at ten percent will reveal the answer. The compound factors are contained in Exhibit 7-5.

Year Deposited				Years	Compound Factor (@10%)	Future Value of $1,000
1	2	3	4			
1,000				→ 1	1.331	$1,331
	1,000			→ 2	1.210	1,210
		1,000		→ 3	1.100	1,100
			1,000	→ 4	1.000	1,000
				Total	4.641	$4,641

The above calculations indicate several points. First, the nursing home will have $4,641 available at the end of the fourth year if deposits of $1,000 are made at the end of each of the four years and each deposit earns ten percent. Second, the compound factors in Exhibit 7-5 are for the number of years the money is invested. The $1,000 deposit made at the end of the first year will be compounded the second year, the third year, and the fourth year. The second year deposit will be compounded the third year and the fourth year. The third year deposit will be compounded the fourth year, and the final deposit made at the end of the fourth year will not be compounded at all since it has no time to earn any return. Third, as before, when the payments are equal in each year, the sum of the individual compound factors can be applied and multiplied by the payment amount. In the case above, $1,000 could be multiplied by 4.641. Exhibit 7-6 gives a table with these values already calculated.

METHODS OF EVALUATION

This section will discuss and illustrate the use of three commonly employed methods of evaluating capital expenditure and capital financing alternatives. Each of these methods is classified as a discounted cash flow technique. This simply means that each employs the time value of money concept. Each method is useful in evaluating a specific type of capital expenditure or capital financing alternative. Specifically, the three methods and their areas of application are—

Method of Evaluation	Application
Net Present Value	Capital Financing Alternatives
Profitability Index	Capital Expenditures with Financial Benefits
Equivalent Annual Cost	Capital Expenditures with Non Financial Benefits

Net Present Value

A net present value analysis is a very useful way to analyze alternative methods of capital financing. In most situations, the objective in this particular type of decision is very clear: the commodity being dealt with is money and it is management's goal to minimize the cost of financing operations. We will discuss shortly how this goal may conflict with solvency when the effects of cost reimbursement are considered.

Net present value simply equals the discounted cash inflows less the discounted cash outflows. In a comparison of two alternative financing packages, the one with the highest net present value should be selected.

The lease example described earlier illustrates this concept. Assume that the asset in question can be financed with a four year annual $1,000 lease payment or purchased outright for $2,800. Assume that the discount rate is ten percent, which may reflect either the borrowing cost or the investment rate depending upon which alternative is relevant. We know that the present value cost of the lease is $3,169 from our prior analysis. This amount is greater than the present value cost of the purchase which is $2,800. With no consideration given to cost reimbursement, the purchase alternative is the lowest cost alternative method of financing.

However, for accuracy the effects of cost reimbursement should be considered. Reimbursement of costs would mean that the facility would be entitled to reimbursement for depreciation if the asset were purchased, or the rent payment if the asset were leased. (Some third party cost payers limit reimbursement on leases to depreciation and interest if the lease is treated as an installment purchase.) Assuming that straight line depreciation is use, and that 80% of expenses are reimbursed by third party cost payers, the present value of the reimbursed cash inflow using the discount factors from Exhibit 7-4 would be as follows:

	Annual Reimburse- ment	Discount Factor	% of Cost Reimburse- ment	
Present Value of Reimbursed Depreciation =	$\dfrac{\$2800}{4}$ ×	3.169 ×	.80	= $1775
Present Values of Reimbursed Lease Payments =	$1000 ×	3.169 ×	.80	= $2536

If the asset were purchased, the organization would pay out $2800 immediately. However, for each of the next four years it would be reimbursed for the noncash expense item of depreciation in the amount of $700 per year ($2800/4). However, since only 80% of the patients are cost payers only $560 per year would be received (.8 x $700). If the asset were leased, the organization would be permitted reimbursement of the lease payment in the amount of $1,000 per year. However, since only 80% of the patients are covered by cost formulas, only $800 (.80 × $1000) would be paid.

The net present value of these two financing alternatives considering cost reimbursement would be as follows:

		Present Value of Reimbursement (Cash Inflows)	Present Value of Payments (Cash Outflows)	Net Present Value
Net Present Value Of Purchase	=	1775	-$2800	=	-1025
Net Present Value Of Lease	=	2536	-$3169	=	- 633

In this specific case, cost reimbursement has changed the relative
desirability of the two financing alternatives. If the organization's objective is cost minimization, then the purchase alternative should be
selected, since the present value of costs are lower under this alternative. If, however, the organization is primarily interested in solvency, then the effect of cost reimbursement should be considered, and the
lease alternative becomes the best financing package.

Profitability Index

The profitability index is another example of a discounted cash flow
method of capital project evaluation. It is of primary importance in
cases where the benefits of the projects are mostly financial, for example a capital project that saves costs or expands revenue with a
primary purpose of increased profits. In these situations, there is
usually a constraint on the availability of funding. Thus, those projects with the highest rate of return per dollar of capital investment are
the best candidates for selection. The profitabiliy index attempts to
compare rates of return. The numerator is the net present value of the
project and the denominator is the investment cost.

$$\text{Profitability Index} = \frac{\text{Net Present Value}}{\text{Investment Cost}}$$

To illustrate the use of this measure, let's assume that a hospital is
considering an investment in a shared laundry with a group of
neighboring hospitals. The initial investment cost would be $10,000
for the purchase of new equipment and delivery trucks. Savings in
operating costs are estimated to be $2,000 per year for the entire ten-

year life of the project. If the discount rate is again assumed to be 10%, the following calculations could be made, ignoring the effect of cost reimbursement and using the discount factors of Exhibit 7-4.

$$\text{Present Value of Operating Savings} = \$2,000 \times 6.145 = \$12,290$$

$$\text{Net Present Value} = \$12,290 - \$10,000 = \$2,290$$

$$\text{Profitability Index} = \frac{\$2,290}{\$10,000} = .229$$

Values for profitability indexes that are greater than zero imply that the project is earning at a rate greater than the discount rate. Given no funding constraints, all projects with profitability indexes greater than zero should be funded. However, in most situations funding constraints do exist and only a portion of those projects with profitability indexes greater than zero are actually accepted.

The above calculations give no consideration to the effects of cost reimbursement. If we assume that 80% of the facilities expenses are reimbursed then the following additional calculations must be made.

$$\text{Present Value of Reimbursed Depreciation} = \frac{\$10,000}{10} \times 6.145 \times .80 = \$4,916$$

$$\text{Present Value of Lost Reimbursement from Operating Savings} = \$2,000 \times 6.145 \times .80 = \$9,832$$

$$\text{Net Present Value} = \$2,290 + \$4,916 - \$9,832 = -\$2,626$$

$$\text{Profitability Index} = \frac{-2626}{10,000} = -.2626$$

The above calculations require some clarification. We are adjusting the initially calculated net present value of $2,290 to reflect the effects of cost reimbursement. Depreciation is the first item to be considered. Since we have 80% of our patients on cost reimbursement formulas, we can expect to receive 80% of the annual depreciation charge of $1,000 ($10,000/10) or $800 per year as a reimbursement cash flow. The present value of this stream is $4,916 and is added to the initial net present value of $2,290. The second item to be considered is the operating savings. If this investment is undertaken, we anticipate a yearly savings of $2,000 for the next ten years. However, that savings will reduce our reimbursable costs by $2,000 annually and will mean that 80% of that amount or $1,600 will be lost annually in reimbursement. The present value of that loss for the ten years is $9,832 and is subtracted from the initial net present value. The effect of cost reimbursement will thus reduce increased costs associated with new programs, but it will also reduce the cost savings associated with new programs.

As in our earlier lease example, a conflict may exist when cost reimbursement is considered. On one hand, the project offers a substantial return in the form of reduced operating costs. However, because of the nature of reimbursement for capital costs in cost reimbursement formulas, the project is not profitable. This lack of profitability may threaten the solvency of the facility if the shared laundry project is accepted.

Equivalent Annual Cost

Equivalent annual cost is the last discounted cash flow method of evaluation that we will discuss. It is of primary value in the selection of capital projects where alternatives exist. Usually these are capital expenditure projects that are classified as operational continuance or other (see page 151). The profitability index measure just discussed is used for those projects where the benefits are primarily financial in nature.

Equivalent annual cost is the expected average cost considering both capital and operating cost over the life of the project. It is calculated by dividing the sum of the present value of operating costs over the life of the project and the present value of the investment cost by the discount factor for an annualized stream of equal payments which is presented in Exhibit 7-4.

$$\text{Equivalent Annual Cost} = \frac{\text{Present Value of Operating Cost} + \text{Present Value of Investment Cost}}{\text{Present Value of Annuity (Exhibit 7-4)}}$$

To illustrate use of this measure, assume that an extended care facility must invest in a sprinkler system to maintain its license. After investigation, two alternatives are identified. One sprinkler system would require a $5,000 investment and an annual maintenance cost of $500 in each year of its estimated ten-year life. An alternative sprinkler system can be purchased for $10,000 that would require only $200 in maintenance cost each year of its estimated twenty-year life

Ignoring cost reimbursement and assuming a discount factor of ten percent, the following calculations can be made.

Equivalent Annual Cost
($5,000 Sprinkler System)

$$\text{Present Value of Operating Costs} = \$500 \times 6.145 = \$3,073$$

$$\text{Present Value of Investment} = \$5,000$$

$$\text{Equivalent Annual Cost} = \frac{\$3,073 + \$5,000}{6.145} = \$1,314$$

Equivalent Annual Cost
($10,000 Sprinkler System)

$$\text{Present Value of Operating Costs} = \$200 \times 8.514 = \$1,703$$

$$\text{Present Value of Investment} = \$10,000$$

$$\text{Equivalent Annual Cost} = \frac{\$1,703 + \$10,000}{8.514} = \$1,375$$

From this analysis, the $5,000 sprinkler system would produce the lowest equivalent annual cost, $1,314 per year when compared to the $1,375 equivalent annual cost of the $10,000 system. Two points should be made with respect to this analysis. First, the equivalent annual cost method permits comparison of two alternative projects with different lives. In this case a ten-year life project was compared to a project with a twenty-year life. However, there is an assumption that the technology will not change and that in ten years the relevant alternatives will still be the two systems analyzed. In situations of estimated rapid technology changes, some subjective weight should be given to projects of shorter duration. In the above example, this is no problem, since the project with the shorter life also has the lowest equivalent annual cost. Second, equivalent annual cost is not identical to the reported or accounting cost. The annual reported accounting cost for these two alternatives would be the annual depreciation expenses plus the maintenance cost.

$$\text{Accounting Expense Per Year ($5,000 sprinkler system)} = \frac{\$5,000}{10}$$

$$+ \$500 = \$1,000$$

$$\text{Accounting Expense Per Year ($10,000 sprinkler system)} = \frac{\$10,000}{20}$$

$$+ \$200 = \$700$$

Relying on information like the above that does not incorporate the time value concept of money can produce misleading results, as it does in this example. The second alternative is not the lowest cost alternative when the cost of capital is included. In this case, the savings of $5,000 in investment cost between the two systems can be used either to generate additional investment income or to reduce outstanding indebtedness. It is assumed that the appropriate discount rate for each of these two alternatives would be 10%.

Once again, the effects of cost reimbursement should be considered. When they are, again assuming that 80% of the hospital's accounting costs are reimbursed; the following series of calculations result.

Equivalent Annual Cost
($5,000 sprinkler system)

Present Value of
Reimbursed Operating $\quad = \quad \$500 \times 6.145 \times .80 = \$2458$
  Costs

Present Value of
Reimbursed $\qquad = \quad \dfrac{\$5,000}{10} \times 6.145 \times .80 = \$2,458$
Depreciation

Equivalent Annual Cost $= \quad \$1314 - \dfrac{(\$2458 + \$2458)}{6.145} = \$514$

Equivalent Annual Cost
($10,000 sprinkler system)

Present Value of
Reimbursed Operating $\quad = \quad \$200 \times 8.514 \times .8 = \$1362$
  Costs

Present Value of
Reimbursed
Depreciation $= \dfrac{\$10,000}{20} \times 8.514 \times .8 = \$3406$

Equivalent Annual Cost $= \$1375 - \dfrac{(\$1362 + \$3406)}{8.514} = \$815$

Once again, some clarification of the above calculations may be useful. To reflect the effect of cost reimbursement, consideration must be given to the reimbursement of reported expenses under the two alternative sprinkler systems. The reported expense items for both sprinkler systems are depreciation and maintenance cost, which is referred to as an operating cost. Depreciation for the $5,000 sprinkler system will be $500 per year ($500/10) and 80% of this amount, $400, will be reimbursed each year. The present value of the reimbursed depreciation ($400 × 6.145) is $2,458. Using the same procedure the present value of reimbursed depreciation for the $10,000 sprinkler system is $3,406 ($400 × 8.514). In a similar fashion the maintenance costs for these two sprinkler systems will also be reimbursed. For the $5,000 system, the annual $500 maintenance cost will yield $400 in new reimbursement (.80 × $500) per year. The present value of this reimbursement inflow is $2,458. Using the same calculations for the $10,000 sprinkler system yields a present value of $1,362. Both the present value of reimbursed depreciation and maintenance costs are then annualized and subtracted from the initially calculated equivalent annual cost to derive new equivalent annual costs that reflect cost reimbursement effects.

In this case, cost reimbursement did not change the decision. The lower cost sprinkler system, after consideration of the effects of reimbursement, is still the best alternative. In fact, the relative difference has increased.

SOURCES OF FINANCING

The health care industry has experienced an explosive rate of growth in the last several decades. In 1974, expenditures for just new hospital construction exceeded $4 billion. This growth in capital assets has required significant amounts of financing. The major categories of financing capital assets in the health care industry are—

- government
- prior reserves
- contributions
- debt

Exhibit 7-7 illustrates the changing pattern in sources of financing in the hospital industry. There is an increasing reliance upon debt financing to meet capital financing needs. This trend has been continuing for some time and is not likely to change in the near future.

With this increase, there is a need to understand the nature of debt financing in the health care industry. Specifically, decision makers need to know the important factors in assessing the alternative sources of financing, the specific alternative sources of financing available and the mechanics of financing arrangements.

Characteristics of Capital Financing Sources

There are a number of factors that effect the relative desirability of alternative sources of debt financing. The most important may be classified into the following five categories:

1. cost
2. risk
3. adequacy
4. availability
5. effect on other sources

Cost

Cost is not as easily determined as might be imagined. You cannot simply compare interest rates and necessarily infer that the financial package with the lowest interest rate is the lowest cost financing source. Major elements of cost would be interest, reserve requirements and front end fees.

Interest is a pretty obvious component of cost and needs little explanation, however reserve requirements and front end fees do. Reserve requirements force the borrower to set aside some money to be used for normal debt service or to meet some contingency. The availability of this reserve fund reduces the risk to the lendors: the presence of a reserve requirement reduces the amount of money effectively borrowed and thus increases the effective interest cost. Front end fees include such things as—

- underwriter's fees
- feasibility study costs
- legal fees
- printing fees
- application costs
- yield adjustment points

Front end fees also reduce the amount of money actually received in a loan and thus increase the effective interest cost.

Risk

Risk is a term used to describe how the position of the borrower would be affected given unforseen changes. Two major elements of risks in a debt financing plan are prepayment provisions and repayment schedule.

Prepayment provisions specify what penalty, if any, will be charged for early retirement of the debt. The penalty is usually stated as a percentage of the principal or par value of the outstanding indebtedness. It represents a risk factor because a reduction in general interest rates or an improvement in the financial condition of the borrower may justify a reduced interest rate. However, the penalty for prepayment limits the economic advantage of early prepayment and thus increases risk.

Repayment schedules determine the amounts of principal that must be repaid and at what point in time. Early retirement of debt, i.e. shorter-term loans, imply more risk. As the length of the loan is decreased, the probability of failing to make timely payment increases, thus the likelihood of default increases, which is a measure of risk.

Adequacy

The ability of a source of financing to meet the borrower's financing needs is called adequacy. Several items are often mentioned as elements of adequacy:

- percentage financing
- interest costs during construction
- refinancing requirements

The percentage of financing available indicates what percentage of the asset value of the proposed project may be financed with a given source of financing. It is an offshoot of the old real estate loan to value ratio. The larger this percentage, the more adequate the source of financing.

During the period of construction, which may be several years for some projects, interest costs are incurred. These costs must be paid and provision for financing made. If a source of financing permits the borrower to include these costs in the loan, the source of financing is deemed more adequate.

Refinancing some outstanding debt may also be a desired objective in a major, new project. Permission from a source of financing for additional borrowing to meet a refinancing requirement also deems the source more adequate.

Availability

Availability refers to the time period required to obtain funding. The shorter the time period to start funding, the more available the source. There are advantages to quick funding, such as lowered construction costs, earlier operations and perhaps a lower interest rate if interest rates are rising.

Effect on Other Sources

Some sources of financing may restrict an organization's ability to use additional debt financing for future projects or they may restrict the use of leasing. For example, additional parity financing permits a borrower to use additional debt to finance future projects only up to the cost of the project. It is a provision that should be written into financial contracts.

Alternative Debt Financing Sources

At the present time there are four major alternative sources of capital financing available to health care facilities:

1. Tax-exempt revenue bonds
2. FHA insured mortgages
3. Public taxable bonds
4. Conventional mortgage financing

Exhibit 7-8 compares these four sources of financing with respect to the factors that affect capital financing desirability just discussed.

Tax-Exempt Revenue Bonds

Tax exempt revenue bonds permit the interest earned on them to be exempt from federal income taxation. The primary security for such loans is usually a pledge of the revenues of the facility seeking the loan, plus a first mortgage on the assets of the facility. If the tax revenue of a government entity is also pledged, these bonds are referred to as "general obligation bonds." Because of the income tax exemption, the interest rates on a tax-exempt bond are usually 1½-2% lower than other sources of financing.

Most tax-exempt revenue bonds are issued by a state or local authority. The health care facility then enters into a lease arrangement with the authority. Title to the assets remains with the authority until the indebtedness is repaid.

FHA Insured Mortgages

This program is sponsored by the Federal Housing Administration (FHA), but initial processing begins in the Department of Health, Education and Welfare (HEW). Through this program, the government provides mortgage insurance for both proprietary and non-proprietary hospitals. This guarantee reduces the risk of a loan for investors and thus lowers the interest rate that a hospital must pay. However, obtaining the appropriate approvals can often be a time-consuming process.

Public Taxable Bonds

Public taxable bonds are issued in much the same way as tax-exempt revenue bonds except there is no indirect issuing authority and no interest income tax exemption. An investment banking firm usually underwrites the loan and markets the issue to individual investors. Interest rates are thus higher on this type of financing than they would be with a tax exempt issue.

Conventional Mortgage Financing

Conventional mortgage financing is usually privately placed with a bank, pension fund, savings and loan, life insurance company or real estate investment trust. This source of financing can usually be quickly arranged, but does not provide as large a percentage of the total financing requirements for large projects. Thus, greater amounts of equity must be contributed.

Parties Involved

Exhibit 7-9 provides a schematic representation of the parties involved and their relationship in issuing a public tax-exempt revenue bond. This schematic could also be used to illustrate the process of issuing a public taxable bond. The only change would be the deletion of the issuing authority and the direct issuance of the bonds by the health care facility. Specific parties in a bond financing which we shall discuss include—

- issuing authority
- investment banker
- health care facility
- market
- trustee bank
- feasibility consultant
- legal counsel
- bond rating agency

Issuing Authority. Only in tax-exempt financing is the issuing authority involved. In most cases the issuing authority is some state or local governmental authority that may be specially created for the sole purpose of issuing revenue bonds. The issuing authority merely serves as a conduit between the health care facility and the investment banker. In a public taxable issue or in a situation where tax-exempt revenue bonds might be issued directly by the health care facility, the role of the issuing authority may be eliminated.

Investment Banker. In a public or private issue, investment bankers have a dual role. First, they serve as advisors to the health care facility issuing the bonds. In many circumstances, they are the focal point for coordinating the services of the feasibility consultant, legal counsel and bond rating agencies. Their advice can be extremely important in the realization of timely funding under favorable conditions. Second, investment bankers serve as brokers between the market and the issuer of the bond. If investment bankers underwrite the issue, it means that they technically buy the entire issue and are at risk for the sale of these bonds to individual investors. If investment bankers place the issue on a "best efforts basis," they do not purchase the issue and any unsold bonds become the property of the issuer.

Health Care Facility. It is the health care facility that is ultimately the beneficiary of the bond issue. It is also the health care facility that is responsible for repayment of the loan principal. The financial condition of the health care facility and its ability to repay the indebtedness are thus the central concerns of the investor. To provide evidence of the financial condition and risk of the investment to the market, the health care facility usually employs independent consultants to assess various aspects of the facility. The feasibility consultant, legal counsel and bond rating agencies are among these.

Market. The market may consist of a large number of individual investors or a small number of large institutional investors for any given bond issue. In any case, the market purchases the bonds of the issuer with the expectation of some stated rate of return. The market also wants assurances that the bonds will be repaid on a timely basis and that there is not an unreasonable amount of risk.

Trustee Bank. A trustee bank serves as the market's agent once the bonds are sold. Typically, the trustee bank is a commercial bank, in some cases the same bank with which the health care facility has its accounts. The trustee bank may receive the proceeds from the sale of the issue and deliver these monies directly to the hospital or to the contractor as needed. The trustee bank also receives the debt service payments from the health care facility and distributes these to the market or investors. It may also retire outstanding bonds according to a prearranged schedule of retirement and hold additional reserve requirements deposited by the health care facility. Finally, the trustee bank insures that the health care facility is adhering to provisions stated in the bond contract or indenture, such as adequate debt service coverage and working capital positions.

Feasibility Consultant. The feasibility consultant is usually an independent CPA who may or may not be the health care facility's outside auditor. The feasibility consultant's primary function is to assess the financial feasibility of the project and the ability of the health care facility to meet the associated indebtedness. Financial projections for a five-year period are usually made. These projections provide a basis for the investor and the bond rating agency to assess the risk of default.

Legal Counsel. Legal opinion is needed for several reasons. First, in a tax-exempt revenue bond issue, the market is concerned with the legality of the tax exemption. If the interest payments are not determined to be tax-exempt by the Internal Revenue Service, the investors have suffered a significant loss. Second, legal opinion is also necessary to insure that the security pledged by the health care facility, whether it be revenue or assets, is legal and enforceable.

Bond Rating Agencies. Moody's and Standard & Poors are the two primary bond rating agencies, although other smaller ones exist. Their function is to assess the relative risk associated with a given bond issue. They have developed a detailed coding of a risk. This coding is presented in Exhibit 7-10. The bond rating received is an important factor for several reasons. There is a correlation between the interest rate that an issuer must pay and the bond rating associated with that issue. Generally speaking the higher the bond rating the lower the interest rate. For example, a bond rated AAA by Standard & Poors would be likely to have a much lower rate of interest than one rated BBB. In addition, issues below BBB for Standard & Poors or Baa for Moody's are not classified as investment grade. Many institutional investors are prohibited from investing in bonds which carry a rating lower than investment grade. Thus the market for these issues is likely to be thin.

SUMMARY

The capital decision-making process in the health care industry is very complex and involves a large number of independent decision makers. This chapter discussed the process and focused on methods for evaluating capital projects. While not all capital expenditure decisions in the health care industry are decided exclusively on the basis of financial criteria, most consider financial factors important. Three discounted cash flow methods were discussed and their appropriateness illustrated by examples. The chapter concluded with a discussion of the sources of financing in the health care industry, the relative criteria for evaluating alternative sources and the definition of various parties' roles in the issuance of debt financing.

Exhibit 7-1 Capital Decision-Making Parties

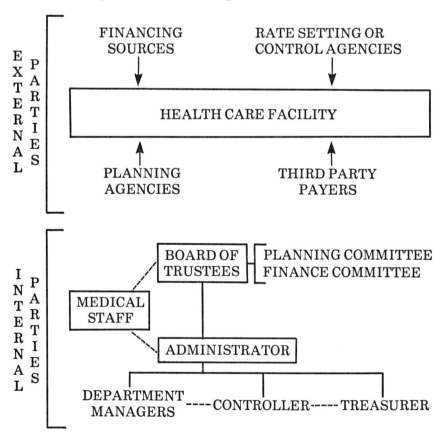

Exhibit 7-2 Review Process of Capital Expenditures Section 1122 of Society Security Act

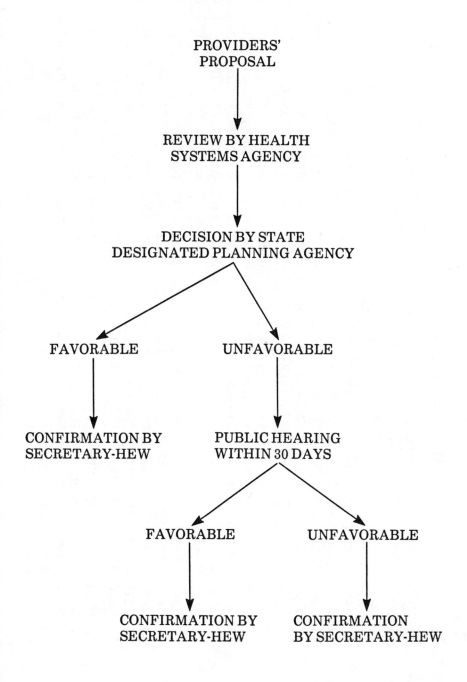

Exhibit 7-3   Present Value of $1.00 Due in N Years

YEARS	4%	6%	8%	10%	12%	14%	16%	18%	20%	22%	24%	26%	28%	30%	40%
1	0.962	0.943	0.926	0.909	0.893	0.877	0.862	0.847	0.833	0.820	0.806	0.794	0.781	0.769	0.714
2	0.925	0.890	0.857	0.826	0.797	0.769	0.743	0.718	0.694	0.672	0.650	0.630	0.610	0.592	0.510
3	0.889	0.840	0.794	0.751	0.712	0.675	0.641	0.609	0.579	0.551	0.524	0.500	0.477	0.455	0.364
4	0.855	0.792	0.735	0.683	0.636	0.592	0.552	0.516	0.482	0.451	0.423	0.397	0.373	0.350	0.260
5	0.822	0.747	0.681	0.621	0.567	0.519	0.476	0.437	0.402	0.370	0.341	0.315	0.291	0.269	0.186
6	0.790	0.705	0.630	0.564	0.507	0.456	0.410	0.370	0.335	0.303	0.275	0.250	0.227	0.207	0.133
7	0.760	0.665	0.583	0.513	0.452	0.400	0.354	0.314	0.279	0.249	0.222	0.198	0.178	0.159	0.095
8	0.731	0.627	0.540	0.467	0.404	0.351	0.305	0.266	0.233	0.204	0.179	0.157	0.139	0.123	0.068
9	0.703	0.592	0.500	0.424	0.361	0.308	0.263	0.225	0.194	0.167	0.144	0.125	0.108	0.094	0.048
10	0.676	0.558	0.463	0.386	0.322	0.270	0.227	0.191	0.162	0.137	0.116	0.099	0.085	0.073	0.035
11	0.650	0.527	0.429	0.350	0.287	0.237	0.195	0.162	0.135	0.112	0.094	0.079	0.066	0.056	0.025
12	0.625	0.497	0.397	0.319	0.257	0.208	0.168	0.137	0.112	0.092	0.076	0.062	0.052	0.043	0.018
13	0.601	0.469	0.368	0.290	0.229	0.182	0.145	0.116	0.093	0.075	0.061	0.050	0.040	0.033	0.013
14	0.577	0.442	0.340	0.263	0.205	0.160	0.125	0.099	0.078	0.062	0.049	0.039	0.032	0.025	0.009
15	0.555	0.417	0.315	0.239	0.183	0.140	0.108	0.084	0.065	0.051	0.040	0.031	0.025	0.020	0.006
16	0.534	0.394	0.292	0.218	0.163	0.123	0.093	0.071	0.054	0.042	0.032	0.025	0.019	0.015	0.005
17	0.513	0.371	0.270	0.198	0.146	0.108	0.080	0.060	0.045	0.034	0.026	0.020	0.015	0.012	0.003
18	0.494	0.350	0.250	0.180	0.130	0.095	0.069	0.051	0.038	0.028	0.021	0.016	0.012	0.009	0.002
19	0.475	0.331	0.232	0.164	0.116	0.083	0.060	0.043	0.031	0.023	0.017	0.012	0.009	0.007	0.002
20	0.456	0.312	0.215	0.149	0.104	0.073	0.051	0.037	0.026	0.019	0.014	0.010	0.007	0.005	0.001

Exhibit 7-3 continued

YEARS	4%	6%	8%	10%	12%	14%	16%	18%	20%	22%	24%	26%	28%	30%	40%
21	0.439	0.294	0.199	0.135	0.093	0.064	0.044	0.031	0.022	0.015	0.011	0.008	0.006	0.004	0.001
22	0.422	0.278	0.184	0.123	0.083	0.056	0.038	0.026	0.018	0.013	0.009	0.006	0.004	0.003	0.001
23	0.406	0.262	0.170	0.112	0.074	0.049	0.033	0.022	0.015	0.010	0.007	0.005	0.003	0.002	
24	0.390	0.247	0.158	0.102	0.066	0.043	0.028	0.019	0.013	0.008	0.006	0.004	0.003	0.002	
25	0.375	0.233	0.146	0.092	0.059	0.038	0.024	0.016	0.010	0.007	0.005	0.003	0.002	0.001	
26	0.361	0.220	0.135	0.084	0.053	0.033	0.021	0.014	0.009	0.006	0.004	0.002	0.002	0.001	
27	0.347	0.207	0.125	0.076	0.047	0.029	0.018	0.011	0.007	0.005	0.003	0.002	0.001	0.001	
28	0.333	0.196	0.116	0.069	0.042	0.026	0.016	0.010	0.006	0.004	0.002	0.002	0.001	0.001	
29	0.321	0.185	0.107	0.063	0.037	0.022	0.014	0.008	0.005	0.003	0.002	0.001	0.001	0.001	
30	0.308	0.174	0.099	0.057	0.033	0.020	0.012	0.007	0.004	0.003	0.002	0.001	0.001	0.001	
40	0.208	0.097	0.046	0.022	0.011	0.005	0.003	0.001	0.001						

Exhibit 7-4   Present Value of $1.00 Received Annually for N Years

YEARS	4%	6%	8%	10%	12%	14%	16%	18%	20%	22%	24%	25%	26%	28%	30%	40%
1	0.962	0.943	0.926	0.909	0.893	0.877	0.862	0.847	0.833	0.820	0.806	0.800	0.794	0.781	0.769	0.714
2	1.886	1.833	1.783	1.736	1.690	1.647	1.605	1.566	1.528	1.492	1.457	1.440	1.424	1.392	1.361	1.224
3	2.775	2.673	2.577	2.487	2.402	2.322	2.246	2.174	2.106	2.042	1.981	1.952	1.923	1.868	1.816	1.589
4	3.630	3.465	3.312	3.170	3.037	2.914	2.798	2.690	2.589	2.494	2.404	2.362	2.320	2.241	2.166	1.849
5	4.452	4.212	3.993	3.791	3.605	3.433	3.274	3.127	2.991	2.864	2.745	2.689	2.635	2.532	2.436	2.035
6	5.242	4.917	4.623	4.355	4.111	3.889	3.685	3.498	3.326	3.167	3.020	2.951	2.885	2.759	2.643	2.168
7	6.002	5.582	5.206	4.868	4.564	4.288	4.039	3.812	3.605	3.416	3.242	3.161	3.083	2.937	2.802	2.263
8	6.733	6.210	5.747	5.335	4.968	4.639	4.344	4.078	3.837	3.619	3.421	3.329	3.241	3.076	2.925	2.331
9	7.435	6.802	6.247	5.759	5.328	4.946	4.607	4.303	4.031	3.786	3.566	3.463	3.366	3.184	3.019	2.379
10	8.111	7.360	6.710	6.145	5.650	5.216	4.833	4.494	4.192	3.923	3.682	3.571	3.465	3.269	3.092	2.414
11	8.760	7.887	7.139	6.495	5.988	5.453	5.029	4.656	4.327	4.035	3.776	3.656	3.544	3.335	3.147	2.438
12	9.385	8.384	7.536	6.814	6.194	5.660	5.197	4.793	4.439	4.127	3.851	3.725	3.606	3.387	3.190	2.456
13	9.986	8.853	7.904	7.103	6.424	5.842	5.342	4.910	4.533	4.203	3.912	3.780	3.656	3.427	3.223	2.468
14	10.563	9.295	8.244	7.367	6.628	6.002	5.468	5.008	4.611	4.265	3.962	3.824	3.695	3.459	3.249	2.477
15	11.118	9.712	8.559	7.606	6.811	6.142	5.575	5.092	4.675	4.315	4.001	3.859	3.726	3.483	3.268	2.484
16	11.652	10.106	8.851	7.824	6.974	6.265	5.669	5.162	4.730	4.357	4.033	3.887	3.751	3.503	3.283	2.489
17	12.166	10.477	9.122	8.022	7.120	6.373	5.749	5.222	4.775	4.391	4.059	3.910	3.771	3.518	3.295	2.492
18	12.659	10.828	9.372	8.201	7.250	6.467	5.818	5.273	4.812	4.419	4.080	3.928	3.786	3.529	3.304	2.494
19	13.134	11.158	9.604	8.365	7.366	6.550	5.877	5.316	4.844	4.442	4.097	3.942	3.799	3.539	3.311	2.496
20	13.590	11.470	9.818	8.514	7.469	6.623	5.929	5.353	4.870	4.460	4.110	3.954	3.808	3.546	3.316	2.497

Exhibit 7-4 continued

YEARS	4%	6%	8%	10%	12%	14%	16%	18%	20%	22%	24%	25%	26%	28%	30%	40%
21	14.029	11.764	10.017	8.649	7.562	6.687	5.973	5.384	4.891	4.476	4.121	3.963	3.816	3.551	3.320	2.498
22	14.451	12.042	10.201	8.772	7.645	6.743	6.011	5.410	4.909	4.488	4.130	3.970	3.822	3.556	3.323	2.498
23	14.857	12.303	10.371	8.883	7.718	6.792	6.044	5.432	4.925	4.499	4.137	3.976	3.827	3.559	3.325	2.499
24	15.247	12.550	10.529	8.985	7.784	6.835	6.073	5.451	4.937	4.507	4.143	3.981	3.831	3.562	3.327	2.499
25	15.622	12.783	10.675	9.077	7.843	6.873	6.097	5.467	4.948	4.514	4.147	3.985	3.834	3.564	3.329	2.499
26	15.983	13.003	10.810	9.161	7.896	6.906	6.118	5.480	4.956	4.520	4.151	3.988	3.837	3.566	3.330	2.500
27	16.330	13.211	10.935	9.237	7.943	6.935	6.136	5.492	4.964	4.525	4.154	3.990	3.839	3.567	3.331	2.500
28	16.663	13.406	11.051	9.307	7.984	6.961	6.152	5.502	4.970	4.528	4.157	3.992	3.840	3.568	3.331	2.500
29	16.984	13.591	11.158	9.370	8.022	6.983	6.166	5.510	4.975	4.531	4.159	3.994	3.841	3.569	3.332	2.500
30	17.292	13.765	11.258	9.427	8.055	7.003	6.177	5.517	4.979	4.534	4.160	3.995	3.842	3.569	3.332	2.500
40	19.793	15.046	11.925	9.779	8.244	7.105	6.234	5.548	4.997	4.544	4.166	3.999	3.846	3.571	3.333	2.500

Exhibit 7-5 Future Value of $1.00 Received in N Years

Years	2%	4%	5%	6%	8%	10%
1	1.0200	1.0400	1.0500	1.0600	1.0800	1.1000
2	1.0404	1.0816	1.1025	1.1236	1.1664	1.2100
3	1.0612	1.1249	1.1576	1.1910	1.2597	1.3310
4	1.0824	1.1699	1.2155	1.2625	1.3605	1.4641
5	1.1041	1.2167	1.2763	1.3382	1.4693	1.6105
6	1.1262	1.2653	1.3401	1.4185	1.5869	1.7716
7	1.1487	1.3159	1.4071	1.5036	1.7138	1.9488
8	1.1717	1.3686	1.4775	1.5938	1.8509	2.1436
9	1.1951	1.4233	1.5513	1.6895	1.9990	2.3589
10	1.2190	1.4802	1.6289	1.7908	2.1589	2.5938
11	1.2434	1.5395	1.7103	1.8983	2.3316	2.8532
12	1.2682	1.6010	1.7959	2.0122	2.5182	3.1385
13	1.2936	1.6651	1.8856	2.1329	2.7196	3.4524
14	1.3195	1.7317	1.9799	2.2609	2.9372	3.7976
15	1.3459	1.8009	2.0709	2.3966	3.1722	4.1774
16	1.3728	1.8730	2.1829	2.5404	3.4259	4.5951
17	1.4002	1.9479	2.2920	2.6928	3.7000	5.0545
18	1.4282	2.0258	2.4066	2.8543	3.9960	5.5600
19	1.4568	2.1068	2.5270	3.0256	4.3157	6.1160
20	1.4859	2.1911	2.6533	3.2071	4.6610	6.7276
30	1.8114	3.2434	4.3219	5.7435	10.0627	17.4495
40	2.2080	4.8010	7.0400	10.2857	21.7245	45.2597

Exhibit 7-6 Future Value of $1.00 Received Annually for N Years

Years	2%	4%	5%	6%	8%	10%
1	1.0000	1.0000	1.0000	1.0000	1.0000	1.0000
2	2.0200	2.0400	2.0500	2.0600	2.0800	2.1000
3	3.0604	3.1216	3.1525	3.1836	3.2464	3.3100
4	4.1216	4.2465	4.3101	4.3746	4.5061	4.6410
5	5.2040	5.4163	5.5256	5.6371	5.8666	6.1051
6	6.3081	6.6330	6.8019	6.9753	7.3359	7.7156
7	7.4343	7.8983	8.1420	8.3938	8.9228	9.4872
8	8.5830	9.2142	9.5491	9.8975	10.6366	11.4360
9	9.7546	10.5828	11.0266	11.4913	12.4876	13.5796
10	10.9497	12.0061	12.5779	13.1808	14.4866	15.9376
11	12.1687	13.4864	14.2068	14.9716	16.6455	18.5314
12	13.4121	15.0258	15.9171	16.8699	18.9771	21.3846
13	14.6803	16.6268	17.7130	18.8821	21.4953	24.5231
14	15.9739	18.2919	19.5986	21.0151	24.2149	27.9755
15	17.2934	20.0236	21.5786	23.2760	27.1521	31.7731
16	18.6393	21.8245	23.6575	25.6725	30.3243	35.9503
17	20.0121	23.6975	25.8404	28.2129	33.7502	40.5456
18	21.4123	25.6454	28.1324	30.9057	37.4502	45.6001
19	22.8406	27.6712	30.5390	33.7600	41.4463	51.1601
20	24.2974	29.7781	33.0660	36.7856	45.7620	57.2761
30	40.5681	56.0849	66.4388	79.0582	113.2832	164.4962
40	60.4020	95.0255	120.7998	154.7620	259.0565	442.5974

Exhibit 7-7 Percentage of Capital Funds Used for Hospital Construction by the Sources of Funds[1]

HOSPITAL CLASSIFICATIONS	SOURCES OF FUNDS							
	Government		Philanthropy		Hospital Reserves[2]		Debt	
	1969	1973	1969	1973	1963	1973	1963	1973
Total	32.3	20.9	13.9	9.9	21.7	14.9	32.0	54.3
Federal	100.0	100.0	0.0	0.0	0.0	0.0	0.0	0.0
Nonfederal	30.3	17.9	14.4	10.3	22.3	15.5	33.0	56.3
Long-term	86.6	49.4	4.8	8.9	2.4	2.3	6.2	39.4
Short-term	26.1	15.7	15.1	10.4	23.8	16.4	35.0	57.5
Nongovernmental								
Not-for-profit	16.6	8.3	17.9	11.8	26.0	17.6	39.6	62.3
Investor-owned	.2	4.0	1.1	0.0	36.9	15.7	62.9	80.3
State and Local								
Governmental	65.9	44.5	6.6	5.3	13.8	11.5	13.7	38.7

[1]1969 data based on construction completed in that year; 1973 data are for construction begun in 1973.

[2]Includes equity for investor-owned facilities.

SOURCE: D. Marine and J. Henderson, "Trends in the Financing of Hospital Construction," *Hospitals* (July 1, 1974).

Exhibit 7-8 Comparative Analysis of Long-Term Financing Alternatives for Hospitals

PROGRAM CHARACTERISTICS	CONVENTIONAL MORTGAGE FINANCING	TAX-EXEMPT HOSPITAL REVENUE BONDS	PUBLIC TAXABLE BONDS	FHA INSURED MORTGAGE (with GNMAE guarantee)
Security	First mortgage given to lender; pledge of gross revenues (substantially all hospital assets pledged)	First mortgage given to trustee bank for benefit of bondholders; pledge of gross revenues (substantially all assets pledged)	First mortgage given to trustee bank for benefit of bondholders; pledge of gross revenues (substantially all assets pledged)	First mortgage given to FHA/pledge of gross revenue
Approximate time required to start to funding	2–6 months	4–8 months	4–8 months	7–12 months
Percentage financing available	Usually 70% (depending on amount on assets available to pledge)	Up to 100%	Up to 100% of project costs, up to 2/3 of asset value	Up to 90%
Eligible costs	Covers all costs (except some movable equipment)	Covers all costs	Covers all costs	Includes: interest during construction; financing fees; start-up costs; refinancing
Term of loan	15–20 years	20–30 years	15 years (usually with a balloon payment in 15th year).	25 years subsequent to construction completion

Exhibit 7-8 continued

PROGRAM CHARACTERISTICS	CONVENTIONAL MORTGAGE FINANCING	TAX-EXEMPT HOSPITAL REVENUE BONDS	PUBLIC TAXABLE BONDS	FHA INSURED MORTGAGE (with GNMAE guarantee)
Front-end fees	Financing and loan commitment fees: 2%/$1,000 principal of loan; legal fees: $25,000	Underwriting fee usually 2%–3½%; feasibility study: $40,000–$75,000; legal and printing: ½ of 1% of principal borrowed	Underwriting fee: 2–4% feasibility study: $40,000–$70,000; legal and printing, ½ of 1% of principal borrowed	Financing fee: 2%; filing and inspection: .8% (.5% of construction inspection fee: 15% application fee, and commitment fee) Annual FHA insurance fee, .5%; GNMAE, .14%
Prepayment provisions	No prepayment for 10 years; 5% penalty, declining thereafter	No prepayment for 10 years; usually 3% penalty, declining thereafter	Nominal call premium after 5 years	15% of original financing any year; 3% penalty for anything in excess of 15%, declining 1/8 of 1% per year thereafter.
Required reserves	1. Depreciation deficiency reserve 2. Debt service reserve equal to one year's average principal and interest requirement	1. Depreciation deficiency reserve 2. Debt service reserve equal to one year's average principal and interest requirement	None	1. Depreciation deficiency reserve
Restriction on leasing	3. Yes—to what extent depends on cash flow and earnings test	None	None	None

Exhibit 7-8 continued

PROGRAM CHARACTERISTICS	CONVENTIONAL MORTGAGE FINANCING	TAX-EXEMPT HOSPITAL REVENUE BONDS	PUBLIC TAXABLE BONDS	FHA INSURED MORTGAGE (with GNMAE guarantee)
Additional parity financing	Yes—subject to approval of conventional lender	Yes—subject to meeting earnings test of 100% on average of prior two years' earnings and pro forma coverage of at least 150%	Yes—subject to approval of underwriter	Yes—subject to approval of FHA
Payments made	Monthly	Quarterly	Quarterly	Monthly

SOURCE: The Ohio Company

Exhibit 7-9 Parties Involved in Public Tax-Exempt Revenue Bond
Issue

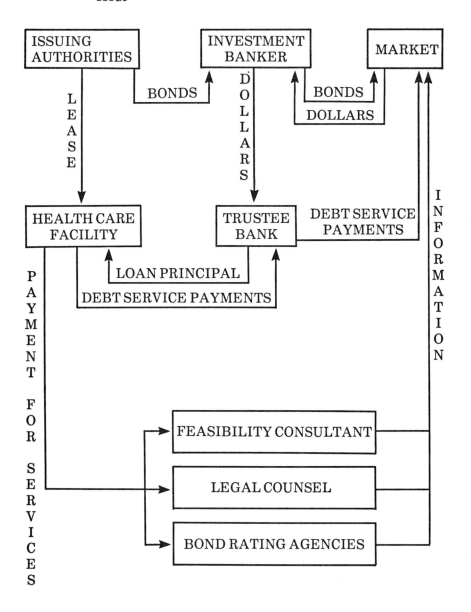

Exhibit 7-10 Bond Ratings

MOODY'S	STANDARD & POOR'S	
Aaa	AAA	INVESTMENT
Aa	AA	GRADE
Al	A+	
A	A	
Baal	BBB+	
Baa	BBB	

Ba	BB	NOT
B	B	INVESTMENT
Caa	CCC	GRADE
Ca	CC	
C	C	

Glossary

Allowable charge: maximum fee allowable by a third party payer for a covered service.

Allowable costs: elements of cost which are reimbursable, usually under a third party reimbursement formula. Typically, allowable costs under Medicare and Medicaid exclude the costs of such things as luxury accommodations, televisions and telephones.

Ambulatory care: all types of health care services delivered on an outpatient basis. This contrasts with services delivered on an inpatient basis or services delivered in the home.

Amortization of debt: process of extinguishing debt through periodic payments which repay the outstanding debt principal.

Ancillary services: services other than room, board and other professional services provided in hospitals or other inpatient health care delivery systems. Examples are radiology, pharmacy and laboratory.

Annual implementation plan (AIP): plan which health system agencies are required to prepare and update annually, describing how they hope to attain long run goals specified in their health systems plan (HSP).

Assignment: agreement by which a patient assigns a hospital or other health care provider the right to receive payment from a third party payer. In most situations, when providers accept assignment from patients, they agree to accept payment from the third party payer as payment in full. This third party payment is generally less than the actual charges billed to patients, especially under Medicare and Medicaid.

Assets: economic potentials, secured by law, from which future benefits are expected to result.

Bad debts: revenue lost by a provider because of patient nonpayment. Medicare limits reimbursement of bad debts to their own patients for covered services.

Bank line of credit: agreement whereby a bank makes funds available to a borrower for a specified period of time, usually one year. Bank lines of credit may or may not be contractually binding upon the bank. A committed line of credit does place a contractual requirement upon the bank to loan funds up to the specified amount.

Best efforts underwriting: relationship with an underwriter whereby the underwriter serves merely as an agent in the sale of bonds and has no commitment to purchase. This contrasts with a firm commitment underwriting arrangement whereby the underwriter agrees to buy the entire issue at a predetermined price.

Blue Cross Association (BCA): organization to which the seventy Blue Cross Plans in the United States belong. Under a contract with the Social Security administration, BCA serves as the intermediary in the Medicare program for approximately 90 per cent of the participating hospitals.

Blue Cross Plan: nonprofit, tax-exempt organization that provides coverage for hospitalization and other health care services on a prepayment basis. Most individual plans are regulated by state insurance commissioners under special enabling legislation. These plans typically provide service benefits rather than indemnity benefits and may pay hospitals on the basis of reasonable costs or charges. The great majority of *Blue Cross Plans* pay institutions on a cost basis.

Blue Shield Plan: nonprofit, tax exempt organization that provides insurance coverage for physicians' services. Coverage is most often sold in conjunction with Blue Cross coverage, although this is not always the case.

Board designated funds: unrestricted funds set aside by the governing board for some designated purpose or purposes.

Bond: debt security, usually issued for long periods of time. Examples are debenture bonds and mortgage bonds.

Book value: amounts at which assets or liabilities are recorded in the accounts. Net book value is usually the assets' cost less any accumulated depreciation.

Budget: detailed plan expressed in financial terms usually for a one-year period. The budget is typically broken down along departmental lines and accounts for both revenue and expense. Hospitals which participate in the Medicare or Medicaid programs are required by law to maintain a one-year operating budget and a three-year capital budget. Section 233 of Public Law 92-603 contains this provision.

Bureau of Health Insurance (BHI): agency within the Social Security administration which administers the Medicare program.

Bureau of Quality Assurance (BQA): agency within the Department of Health, Education and Welfare which administers the Professional Standards Review Organization (PSRO) program.

Capital assets: assets having useful economic lives greater than one year which are not acquired principally for resale. Examples include buildings and equipment. See *fixed assets.*

Capital expenditure review: prospective review of capital expenditure projects of health care facilities to determine the need and appropriateness of the expenditure. The usual initial review agency is the health systems agency. Section 1122 of the Social Security Act requires the state-designated health planning and development agency to serve as the review agency for projects of health care facilities receiving Medicare or Medicaid reimbursement.

Capitation: method of payment for health services in which a provider is paid a fixed per capita amount irrespective of the services provided. This method of payment is characteristic of health maintenance organizations (HMOs).

Cash flow: term usually defined as the summation of net income or excess of revenues over expenses plus depreciation. This quantity provides an index of the availability of cash to meet financial requirements such as amortization of debt and plant replacement.

Catastrophic health insurance: health insurance which provides protection for severe or lengthy illnesses requiring very high treatment costs. Such insurance policies take effect only after some specified minimum expenditure has been reached. Some national health insurance proposals are of this type. Costs for this type of insurance program are generally much lower than those estimated for more comprehensive national health insurance programs.

Catchment area: geographical area defined and serviced by a hospital or other health care facility.

Certificate-of-need: example of capital expenditure review.

Charitable immunity: legal precept used in some states to exclude non-profit or charitable hospitals and other health care facilities from malpractice suits. Exceptions to this doctrine exist; the trend today is towards eliminating the concept of *charitable immunity* for nonprofit health care facilities.

Claims incurred policy: traditional form of malpractice insurance coverage today as contrasted with a claims made policy. In a *claims incurred policy,* the insured is covered for any claims which may arise from an incident that occurred during the policy period. This is true regardless of when the actual claim is made and is limited only by the statute of limitations in the state in which the claim is made.

Claims made policy: alternative form of malpractice insurance coverage to the claims incurred policy. Under this type of insurance arrangement, the insured is covered for any claim made during the policy period, regardless of when the injury may have occurred. Insurance companies contend that a *claims made policy* better enables them to establish more accurate rates. However, there is some transference of risk from the insurer to the insured because many claims for injury will not occur in the policy period.

Coinsurance: cost sharing arrangement whereby an individual assumes a certain percentage of the costs of covered services and the individual's health insurance assumes the remainder.

Community rating: method whereby a health insurer determines the premium required to maintain solvency. In a *community rating* scheme, as contrasted with an experience rated scheme, the premium is based on the average costs of all subscribers in a specific geographical area or industry and does not vary for different groups or subgroups of these subscribers. *Community rating* spreads the cost of illness evenly over all the subscribers and does not charge those who are ill more than those who are healthy.

Coordination of benefits: procedures used by health insurers to avoid duplication of payments for claims made under more than one insurance policy.

Copayment: form of cost sharing whereby the insured pays a specific amount per unit of service received. This differs from a coinsurance arrangement under which payment is expressed as a percentage of cost.

Cost: exchange price paid for goods or services at the time of acquisition. Cost is measured at the date of acquisition by the amount of the cash outlay, the amount of the indebtedness incurred, or the cash equivalent when noncash assets are exchanged.

Cost center: accounting subentity to which all related costs are charged for accounting or reimbursement purposes. In most cases, a cost center usually follows the departmental structure of the organization.

Cost based reimbursement: method of payment used by many third parties based on the actual costs of providing services to the covered patient, not on the charges actually made for those services. There are a variety of cost formulas which specify whether or not a plus factor is allowable and what type of cost apportionment methods may be used. Medicare. Medicaid, most Blue Cross plans and other governmental programs typically reimburse hospitals and other health care facilities on the basis of costs.

Coupon rate of interest: rate of interest stated on the face of a bond certificate, used to determine the amount of periodic interest promised.

Coverage: ratio of cash flow to debt service on bonds. The ratio indicates the relative security of the bond to the investor and affects the credit rating.

Credit rating: index of risk granted a given debt security by an independent credit rating agency, such as Moody's or Standard & Poors. This rating has an impact upon the effective interest rate of the debt security and also its marketability.

Current assets: liquid assets which can be expected to be directly or indirectly converted into cash within one year or the operating cycle of the entity, whichever is longer.

Current liabilities: obligations that fall due and will be paid within one year or the operating cycle of the entity, whichever is longer.

Debenture: debt instrument in which the only protection against non-payment is the general credit of the issuer. This is in contrast to real estate mortgage loans or chattel mortgage loans upon which there is an additional protection of security specified in the mortgage.

Debt service: amount of payment required for interest and amortization of the principal on outstanding bonds due in a defined accounting period.

Deductible: cost sharing arrangement whereby the insured must incur an initial loss or expense of a specified amount within a given time period before the insurer assumes liability for any additional costs of covered services. *Deductibles,* coinsurance and copayment provisions are all examples of cost sharing arrangements whose effect may be a reduction in the demand for health care services on the part of the insured.

Depreciation: depreciation accounting is a system of accounting which distributes the cost or other basic value of tangible capital assets over their estimated useful life in a systematic and rational manner. It is a process of allocation and should not be viewed as one of valuation. Depreciation for any year is a portion of the total cost or basic value that is allocated to that year.

Designated planning agency: See *State health planning and development agency.*

Direct cost: cost which may be directly identified with a specific activity, department or cost center. Such types of cost may be contrasted with indirect cost.

Discount factor: factor used to express the value of dollars received in the future in present dollar terms.

Dual choice: practice of giving individuals an opportunity to select from more than one health insurance or health program to pay for or provide their health services. Under the Health Maintenance Organization Act (Public Law 93-222) employers must provide a dual choice with respect to qualified health maintenance organizations where they are available.

Economic stabilization program: federal program established on August 15, 1971 to control wages and prices. The program was continued in the health care industry until April 1974. The rate of growth in medical care prices during that period showed marked reduction. However, the long-run effectiveness of this control program is still debated.

Economies of scale: cost savings that result from the production of services in larger volumes. There is conflicting evidence on the existence of economies of scale in the hospital industry. Much of this difference relates to the unit of production studied, which has typically been patient days or admissions. When a more homogenous unit of output at the departmental level is examined, *economies of scale* do appear present in the hospital industry. A primary argument for increasing shared service activity relates to the existence of *economies of scale.*

Endowment funds: funds given by a donor who has stipulated that the principal portion must be maintained in perpetuity. Income from investment of these funds may be expended however.

Effective rate of interest: rate of interest determined by dividing the actual cost of borrowing by the amount borrowed for a one-year period. In many cases, this rate will be different than the stated rate of interest if there is a discount or premium on the indebtedness or a required compensating balance.

Excess of revenues over expenses: difference between revenues and expenses for a defined accounting period. This term is used synonomously with *net income*, however, the term *excess of revenues over expenses* is used predominantly in nonprofit hospital industries.

Expense: expired cost incurred directly or indirectly in the earning of revenue.

Experience rating: method used by health insurance companies to determine their premiums, based on the average cost of anticipated health care utilization by various groups and subgroups of subscribers. The premiums calculated will thus vary with the experience of the group and subgroups and will be affected by such variables as age, sex and health status. This method differs from community rating methods.

Extended care facility: term used in Medicare reimbursement to indicate skilled nursing facility which is qualified for participation in the Medicare program. Medicare coverage for extended care services is limited to one hundred days of posthospital care during any spell of illness. These same limitations do not apply to skilled nursing facilities benefits under the Medicaid program.

Factoring: practice of one organization selling its accounts receivable to another organization at a discount. The organization purchasing the accounts receivable assumes full risk for loss if the accounts eventually prove uncollectable. Factoring of accounts receivable in the health care industry is not frequently done. However, some health care facilities have factored Medicaid receivables because of extremely slow payment.

"Fast track" construction: method of scheduling used to shorten the overall time between the decision to construct a building and occupancy. This is accomplished by overlapping programming and design and construction, so that one stage begins before the other is actually completed.

FNMA (Fannie Mae): Federal National Mortgage Association, a federal agency which purchases mortgages insured by the Federal Housing Administration (FHA). This assures a much wider secondary market for these types of securities.

Feasibility study: report of an independent firm of accountants or other consultants which documents an organization's ability to repay prospective debt financing with anticipated cash flow. This document is usually an integral part of the review conducted by bond rating agencies and has a dramatic impact on the credit rating eventually received and thus the effective interest rate. *Feasibility studies* may also be used by health systems agencies and in this context may be broadened to include nonfinancial aspects such as need.

Federal Register: daily publication of the federal government which provides information to the public concerning proposed and final rules, legal notices and other proclamations and orders that have general applicability and legal effect. The *Register* publishes material from all federal agencies.

Finance lease: lease viewed by tax authorities and/or accountants as a conditional sales agreement, preventing the rental amounts paid from becoming the relevant measure of expense associated with the leased asset. The usual cost of ownership and depreciation, plus the financing cost on the lease, become the recognized costs of the asset leased.

Financial requirements: term coined by the American Hospital Association (AHA) to designate the total need for funds by a health care entity. Total financial requirements may be greater or less than the expenses reported for a given accounting period.

Firm commitment underwriting: underwriting arrangement with an investment banker whereby the investment banker agrees to buy the entire issue of bonds at a predetermined price. This contrasts with best efforts underwriting.

Fiscal agents: contractors who process and pay claims on behalf of a state Medicaid agency. These contractors usually assume no risk and simply serve in an administrative capacity for the state.

Fiscal year: twelve-month period for which an annual accounting is made. In many situations this may coincide with the calender year, January 1st to December 31st.

Fund: cash or other assets held separately for a specific purpose such as a pension fund or a bond sinking fund. The contribution of cash or other assets to a fund is sometimes referred to as *funding.* For example, the depositing of cash in an account reserved for plant replacement is sometimes referred to as funding depreciation.

Governing board: controlling board of an organization, having overall responsibility for management. Most members of this board are nonemployees of the organization.

GNMA: Government National Mortgage Association, a federal agency issuing its own securities on the open market. These securities are backed by the yield on federally insured mortgages.

Group practice: formal association of three or more physicians. Income from the practice is usually pooled and redistributed to the individual members according to some prearranged formula. Groups may be single or multi-specialty in nature. A multi-specialty group has the potential to provide continuity of care and integration of services which may be advantageous to its patients.

Health maintenance organizaton (HMO): organization which establishes a contractual relationship with consumers to deliver an agreed upon set of basic and supplemental health maintenance and treatment services. Prepayment for these services is based upon a fixed amount for each person or family unit enrolled in the organization without consideration of the actual services utilized. Some empirical evidence demonstrates that *HMO's* may provide high quality medical services at lower costs because of reductions in the rates for hospitalization and surgery. Some or all of these differences may be attributable to the types of groups enrolled in HMO plans. Under the *Health Maintenance Organization Act* all employers must offer an *HMO* option to their employees whenever a qualified *HMO* exists in the area.

Health systems agencies (HSA): agencies concerned with health planning created under P.L. 93-641. Functions of *HSAs* include preparation of a health system plan and annual implementation plan, issuance of grants and contracts, review and approval or disapproval of proposed uses of federal funds in the *HSA's* health service area and review of proposed, new and existing institutional health services and the making of recommendations with respect to these proposals to the designated state health planning and development agency.

Health system plan: long-run health plan prepared by a health systems agency for its health service area, specifying the goals established by the agency for that area. Section 1513 of the Public Health Service Act specifies the nature of the health system plan.

Home health agency: agency which provides health services to individuals as needed in the home. To be eligible for Medicare reimbursement, these agencies must provide skilled nursing services and at least one additional therapeutic service such as physical therapy, speech therapy or occupational therapy.

Hospital based physician: physician who spends most practice time in one or more hospitals instead of an office setting. Financial arrangements with these physicians are varied and may include salary, percentage of fees and percentage of income.

Hospital insurance program: compulsory portion of Medicare which automatically enrolls all persons over 65 who are entitled to benefits under the Social Security system, others under the age of 65 who are also eligible for benefits because of disability and insured workers and their families who require renal dialysis or kidney transplantation.

Indemnity benefits: health insurance policies which provide benefits in the form of cash payments rather than services. *Indemnity insurance* contracts typically specify maximum amounts that will be paid for a listing of covered services. After the patient has been billed for covered services, the insurance company either remits payment to the patient or directly to the provider. This type of benefit package contrasts with service benefits.

Indirect cost: cost which cannot be directly identified with a specific activity product, or department. *Indirect costs* are usually allocated to direct or revenue departments using some allocation basis.

Intermediary: public or private organization selected by the providers of health care under the hospital insurance program to pay claims and perform administrative functions for the Secretary of Health, Education and Welfare. In most cases, the intermediary is a Blue Cross Plan. However, some hospitals have dropped Blue Cross as their *intermediary* and selected a commercial insurance company.

Intermediate care facility: institution which provides health care related services to individuals who do not require the same degree of care available in a hospital or skilled nursing facility. These institutions are recognized under the Medicaid program and are eligible for reimbursement.

Investment banker: middle-man between the issuer of bonds and the public market. Investment bankers are also known as underwriters when they purchase all of the bonds from the issuer.

Issuer: party who is borrowing money through a sale of bonds, usually the hospital or health care organization. However, in a tax-exempt financing the *issuer* is most often a state or local authority who borrows money on the hospital's behalf.

Joint Commission on Accreditation of Hospitals (JCAH): organization whose purpose is to encourage the attainment of high standards of medical care within the hospital industry. Medical inspectors from the *JCAH* inspect hospitals and issue a Certificate of Accreditation. Accreditation by the *JCAH* has been used by Medicare and other public programs as a condition of participation.

Joint Underwriting Association (JUA): association comprised of insurers who have been authorized by a given state to write a certain kind of insurance within that state. In the malpractice area, these associations have been formed to insure the availability of malpractice insurance.

Lease: contract which grants possession of an asset for a period of time in return for some stated consideration, such as rent.

Legal opinion: written assurance from attorneys that the issuance of bonds complies with any applicable statutes and court decisions and that these bonds are legally enforceable.

Liabilities: debts or obligations of an accounting entity.

Limits on liability: limits on professional liability that may be imposed by state law. Some states have officially enacted legislation that places limits on the dollar amount of malpractice awards. The constitutionality of these laws is questionable.

Long-term care: health care or personal services required by individuals who are chronically ill, aged, disabled or retarded, provided in an institution or home on a long-term basis.

Major medical: insurance whose major purpose is to provide protection for unusually heavy medical expenses that may result from catastrophic illnesses. These policies do not provide first dollar coverage. Instead, they provide benefits when medical expenses have exceeded a defined base amount paid by the insured.

Malpractice: misconduct or lack of ordinary skill in the performance of professional services. A successful claimant must demonstrate that injury occurred and that the injury was negligently caused.

Management information system: term commonly used to describe a data system, generally automated or computerized, which provides information for management decision making.

Marginal cost: change in total cost that results from a one-unit change in the quantity of services provided. This concept of cost is especially relevant in considering the cost implications of expansions or contractions.

Medicaid: health care program for low-income persons that was authorized by Title XIX of the Social Security Act. It is a federally aided program operated and administered by states.

Maturity: date upon which the principal amount of a bond becomes due.

Medical review: review by a team of physicians and other health care personnel required by Medicaid for each individual receiving care in a long-term care facility.

Medicare: nation-wide health insurance program for individuals eligible for social security benefits. The program became effective July 1, 1966 and is often referred to as Title XVIII of the Social Security Act. It contains two separate but coordinated programs: hospital insurance (Part A), and supplementary medical insurance (Part B).

Mortgage bonds: bonds secured by a lien upon real property.

Municipal bonds: bonds issued by states or political subdivisions such as counties, cities or villages. In most cases, interest paid on municipal bonds is exempt from federal income taxation. Tax-exempt bonds and *municipal bonds* are often used interchangeably.

Mutual insurance companies: insurance companies that have no capital stock and instead are owned by the policyholders. Any earnings over and above operating expenses and reserve requirements become the property of the policy holders and are returned to them, usually in the form of dividends or reduced premiums. Some hospitals have formed *mutual insurance companies* to provide malpractice insurance coverage.

Net income: difference between revenue and expenses for a given accounting period. See also *excess of revenues over expenses.*

Nursing differential: differential of 8½ percent of routine inpatient nursing salary costs that is allowed for Medicare beneficiaries. This differential presumably reflects the above average costs that are incurred in providing care to Medicare patients.

Nursing homes: health care facilities which provide nursing care and other personal services to individuals who are not capable of caring for themselves. Nursing homes include the following types of facilities: skilled nursing, intermediate care and extended care.

Opportunity cost: Maximum value that might have been attained if a resource had been used in the next best possible alternative way. Actual dollar costs of resources are usually a valid measure of opportunity cost, however, amortizations of prior expenditures such as depreciation are rarely useful measures of opportunities cost.

Operating lease: sometimes referred to as a true lease in which the lease is not construed to be a transfer of ownership or conditional sale. This type of lease is not capitalized and thus the relevent measure of expense is the periodic rent specified in the lease. This is in contrast to a finance lease.

Outpatient: patient who receives ambulatory care at a health care facility without being admitted to that facility.

Per diem costs: cost per day of care received in an inpatient institution. This figure may be derived by dividing total costs of the institution by the number of inpatient days of care rendered.

Points: one percentage point of the par or principal value of a bond. In the case of a $1,000 bond, a point would be $10.00. Points are merely a method of measuring the value of a bond. They are sometimes referred to as the costs associated with a given financing, e.g., an investment banker may require 2% of the par value of an issue as his fee, or two points.

Prepaid group practice: association of three or more physicians that provides a defined set of services to persons within a given time period in return for a fixed prepayment.

Prevailing charge: charge that is within some normal range of charges most frequently used in a given locality for a stated medical service.

Current Medicare regulations specify the prevailing charge to be the 75th percentile of all customary charges for a specific service by physicians in that area.

Prior authorization: requirement imposed by some third party payers that a provider must justify the need for delivering a service to a patient prior to the actual delivery of that service. Usually prior authorization is limited to the delivery of nonemergency services.

Professional Activity Study (PAS): computerized medical record information system provided by the Commission on Professional Hospital Activities which provides comparative medical record information. For example, periodic reports are delivered to participating hospitals which compare their lengths of stay, numbers and types of tests used and autopsy rates for specifically designated diagnostic conditions with those of other hospitals of similar size and scope of services.

Professional Standards Review Organization (PSRO): physician sponsored organization that has responsibility for reviewing services rendered under the Medicare, Medicaid, and Maternal and Child Health programs. Services rendered to patients under one of these programs and deemed to be medically unnecessary by the *PSRO* organization will not be reimbursed.

Prospective reimbursement: method of reimbursing hospitals or other health care facilities on the basis of rates established in advance of the delivery of the services, and not affected by the amount of actual cost incurred. Medicare, Medicaid and many Blue Cross plans currently reimburse hospitals on a retrospective cost reimbursement basis. An advantage of prospective reimbursement often cited is the potential for improved efficiency and cost reduction that results from the introduction of an incentive on the part of health care facilities to reduce costs.

Prospectus: written document that contains information about an entity which is seeking additional debt or equity financing and information about the terms and purposes of the financing.

Prudent buyer principle: Medicare reimbursement provision that limits reimbursement to a provider for costs in excess of amounts that a prudent and cost conscious buyer would pay.

Public Health Service Act (PHSA): act of Congress which provides legislative authority for federal involvement in health care activities. The Act has been amended many times since its original enactment in 1944. This Act contains authority for involvement in public health programs, biomedical research, health manpower training, family planning, emergency medical services systems, HMO's, regulation of drinking water supplies and health planning and resources development.

Reasonable charge: value defined for Medicare reimbursement of physicians that is the lower of the physicians customary charge for a particular service, or the prevailing charge by physicians for that service in that geographical area. Medicare reimbursement for physician's services is defined to be that value and is thus the lower of the reasonable charge or the actual charge made. For example, assume a physician charges a Medicare patient $100 for a service that he customarily charges $100 for and that the prevailing physician charge for that service (75th percentile) is $80. Medicare would only pay $80.

Reasonable cost: amount stated in most cost reimbursement formulas which third party payers will actually reimburse. *Reasonable cost* of providing covered services is typically modified to limit costs for resources consumed in the production of services to those resources that were necessary for the efficient production of needed services and did not reflect excessive purchase prices under the prudent buyer principle.

Redemption provision: provision included in many bonds allowing issuers at their option to call the bonds, prior to maturity, at a specified price.

Refunding: selling of new debt securities by an issuer to retire outstanding debt securities. The object of refunding or refinancing is usually to reduce interest costs or extend payment of the existing debt.

Reserve fund: special fund established in many bonds to be used for the payment of debt service in the event of a default.

Reserves: balance sheet account established to reflect liabilities faced by insurance companies under existing insurance policies. The process of establishing reserves converts the reporting of expense from a cash to an accrual basis of accounting. Regulatory agencies have some control over the level of reserves maintained.

Retrospective reimbursement: payment to providers by a third party for either costs or charges that have been incurred by subscribers in a prior time period. This contrasts with prospective reimbursement.

Revenue: values received from the furnishing of goods or services.

Revenue bond: bond which is payable exclusively from the revenue generated from the operation of a project. In the case of hospital *revenue bonds,* the gross receipts of the hospital are usually pledged for repayment of the indebtedness. *Revenue bonds* are sometimes referred to as municipal or tax-exempt bonds.

Sale and lease-back: type of transaction in which one party sells an asset to another party and at the same time, leases the asset back from the party to whom the asset was sold.

Security interest: property interest in a debtor's assets which is retained by or conveyed to a creditor as a means of insuring payment.

Self-insure: assumption of risk by an organization against losses.

Serial bonds: issue of bonds where there are different maturities. Serial bonds are usually retired on an equal annual basis or on a level debt service basis. They may be contrasted with term bonds.

Service benefits: insurance benefits whereby payment is made directly to the provider for covered services provided to subscribers. Service benefits may be contrasted with indemnity benefits.

Shared services: formal arrangement whereby two or more hospitals or other health care facilities agree to share the responsibility for the provision of certain medical or nonmedical services. Common examples of shared services are laundry, dietary, and laboratory.

Sinking fund: accumulation of monies in accordance with terms specified in an indebtedness to be used for the eventual retirement of the indebtedness.

Skilled nursing facility (SNF): type of facility defined in Medicare and Medicaid provisions as an institution or a distinct part of another institution which has a transfer arrangement with one or more participating hospitals and which meets other specified conditions. *SNFs* provide a higher level of care than that available in an intermediate care facility and in many Medicaid formulas are allowed a higher rate of reimbursement. Medicare does not reimburse intermediate care facilities.

State health planning and development agency (SHPDA): designated state agency required under Section 1521 of the Public Health Service Act which was created by Public Law 93-641. This agency will serve as the designated review agency for capital expenditure review and administration of the certificate of need program.

Subordinated debt: debt which has provisions that limit the availability of a debtors assets in the event of default. Usually, assets remaining after the satisfaction of all other creditors' claims, including those of general unsecured creditors, may be used for the repayment of subordinated debt in the event of bankruptcy.

Supplementary medical insurance program (SMI): voluntary program of Medicare in which all persons eligible for the hospital insurance program may enroll. This program is financed by payments from enrollees and matching amounts from general federal revenue. Covered services include physicians' services, home health care services, outpatient hospital services, laboratory, pathology, radiology and other health services.

Surgi-center: health care facility which provides surgical treatment to patients on an outpatient basis.

Third party payer: organization that pays for or insures health or medical expenses on behalf of its beneficiaries or subscribers. Third party payers would include Blue Cross, Blue Shield, commercial insurance companies, Medicare and Medicaid.

Title V: title of the Social Security Act that provides the legislative authority for the Maternal and Child Health Care Program.

Title XVIII: title of the Social Security Act which provides the legislative authority for the Medicare program.

Title XIX: title of the Social Security Act which provides the legislative authority for the Medicaid program.

Tax-exempt bonds: bonds upon which the interest is exempt from federal income taxation.

Term bond: bond issue which has only one maturity. It is possible that at certain intervals some of the term bonds may be called and retired through monies set aside in a sinking fund. In most situations, serial bonds, and term bonds are combined in an issue.

Trustee: usually a bank designated as the custodian of funds and the official representative for bond holders.

Underwriter: one or more investment bankers who will purchase and market an entire debt issue for the issuing entity. There is a fee referred to as the underwriting spread which is retained by the underwriter for this service.

Underwriting spread: difference between the price paid by the public for bonds and the price paid to the issuer by the underwriter for those same bonds.

Uniform cost accounting: use of a common set of accounting definitions, procedures, terms and methods for the accumulation and communication of quantitative data that relate to the financial activities of several entities. Most states that have established rate-setting commissions also require *uniform cost accounting* or uniform reporting as a prerequisite to their establishment.

Unrestricted funds: funds which have no third party restriction placed upon their utilization and can be used for any legitimate purpose specified by the governing board.

Usual, customary and reasonable charges: a physician's charges for services that do not exceed the usual charge, the customary charge by other physicians for the same service in the area, or reasonableness. Usual, customary and reasonable charges are similar but not identical to the customary and prevailing charges concept used by Medicare. Most private health insurance plans, except for a few Blue Shield plans, use this approach.

Utilization review: evaluation of the necessity, appropriateness and efficiency of medical services, procedures and facilities. Medicare and Medicaid require, as a condition of participation in the program, that hospitals maintain a special committee to perform a *utilization review* function.

Working capital: investment of an institution in current assets such as cash, marketable securities, accounts receivable and inventories. Net *working capital* is usually defined as the excess of current assets over current liabilities. It is a financial requirement that is usually not recognized in most cost reimbursement formulas.

Workmen's compensation programs: mandatory state social insurance programs that provide cash benefits to workers and their dependents who are disabled as a result of their employment. Medical services are usually covered under these programs.

Yield: actual percentage return to the investor. In many cases, this may be different than the actual coupon rate of interest because the price paid for the bond and the principal value of the bond may be different.

Index

About the Author

William O. Cleverley is Associate Professor, Graduate Program in Hospital and Health Services Administration and Associate Professor of Accounting, College of Administrative Science, at Ohio State University. He edited *Financial Management of Health Care Facilities,* published by Aspen Systems Corporation, and is a frequent contributor to several publications in the health care field. He is the Senior Editor of *Topics in Health Care Financing.* Dr. Cleverley is also a consultant to a number of private and governmental organizations. Dr. Cleverley holds a Ph.D. in Business Administration from the University of California, Berkeley.